P9-CJK-036

Dying at Home

Dying at Home

A Family Guide for Caregiving

Revised and Updated Edition

ANDREA SANKAR

The Johns Hopkins University Press
Baltimore and London

Dying at Home presents first-person accounts related by people who have participated in a home death experience. The accounts are intended to acquaint those who are providing care for someone dying at home with some of the emotions and practical issues involved in this experience. The views expressed in these accounts are not necessarily the views of the author or the publisher. This book is not meant to substitute for medical care of terminally ill persons, and medical treatment should not be based solely on its contents.

Drug dosage: The author and publisher have made reasonable efforts to determine that the selection and dosage of drugs discussed in this text conform to the practices of the general medical community. The medications described do not necessarily have specific approval by the U.S. Food and Drug Administration for use in the diseases and dosages for which they are recommended. In view of ongoing research, changes in governmental regulations, and the constant flow of information relating to drug therapy and drug reactions, the reader is urged to check the package insert of each drug for any change in indications and dosage and for warnings and precautions. This is particularly important when the recommended agent is a new and/or infrequently used drug.

©1991, 1999 The Johns Hopkins University Press
All rights reserved. First edition 1991
Bantam edition 1995
Revised and updated edition 1999
Printed in the United States of America on acid-free paper.
9 8 7 6 5 4 3 2 1

The Johns Hopkins University Press
2715 North Charles Street
Baltimore, Maryland 21218-4363
www.press.jhu.edu

Library of Congress Cataloging-in-Publication Data will be found at the end of this book.
A catalog record for this book is available from the British Library.

ISBN 0-8018-6202-7
ISBN 0-8018-6203-5 (pbk.)

For my mother
Bettyann Horton Sankar
(1918–1987)

Contents

List of Illustrations and Tables xiii

Preface to the Revised Edition xv

Acknowledgments xix

Some Who Died at Home xxi

Introduction 1

Home Death: A Return to Tradition 1

The Term *Caregiver* 2

Factors Contributing to the Trend. 3

    The Desire for Control 3

    The Hospice Movement 4

    The Limitations of Medical Science 4

    Advances in Home-based Technology and Pharmacology 4

    Change in Insurance Reimbursement 5

Problems of Caregiving 5

    The Dying Person 5

    Intimacy 6

    The Caregiver's Responsibility 7

    Physical and Emotional Stamina 10

    Expenses 10

Deciding Whether to Become a Caregiver 11

The Research for This Book 13

    The Method 13

    The Informants 14

How to Read This Book 15

1. Taking the Patient Home to Die 17

Participating in Hospital Care 17

The Appropriateness of Treatment 18

Procedures 19

Bedside Nursing 19

Communicating with the Hospital Staff 21

The Decision to Discharge the Patient 25

Discharge Options 26

Planning the Discharge 27

The Transfer Home 34

Rehospitalization 35

Reasons for Readmission 35

Considering Readmission 39

2. Strangers in the Home:
The Use of Formal Support 42

The Functions of Formal Support 42

To Provide Respite 42

To Provide Skilled Care 43

To Supply Information and Reassurance 44

To Offer Spiritual Support 46

Deciding to Use Formal Support 47

Assessing the Need for Services 50

Types of Agencies 53

Hospice 53

Home Care 58

Health Maintenance Organization 58

Professionals Who Work in the Home 59

Physicians 60

Nurses 62

Home Health Aides 63

Other Professionals 64

Gaining Access to the Formal System 65

Access through Discharge from the Hospital 65

Access without Prior Hospitalization 68

Contacting an Agency 69

Preparations 69

Questions to Ask 69

Finding the Right People 73
Maintaining Privacy: Establishing Boundaries 76

3. Caregiving 79
The Caregiver's Role 79
Problem Solving 80
Decision Making 83
Ethical Dilemmas 85
Conflicts 87
The Dignity and Autonomy of the Dying Person 92
Becoming an Expert 94
The Patient Log 94
The Quality of Life 98

4. Social Support 101
The Meaning of Social Support 102
Types of Support 103
    Support for the Dying Person 104
    Support for the Caregiver 106
    Spiritual Support 108
How the Support System Works 110
    Decision Making 110
    Integrating Support into the Caregiving Routine 111
    Reciprocity 112
    Organizing a Support System 113
The Inclusion of Children 115
Problems in the Support System 118
    When Support Doesn't Work 118
    Lack of Social Support 120

5. The Well-being of the Caregiver 125
Day to Day 125
The Physical Drain 128
The Emotional Strain 131
    Grief 131
    Lack of Control 132

Anger 134

Fear of Death 136

Responsibilities to Others 138

Coping 140

Taking Breaks 141

Social Support 142

Support Groups and Therapy 143

Laughter 144

Making Life Easier 145

Work 146

Spiritual Support 148

What Enabled Caregivers to Care and
What It Meant to Them 148

6. Demystifying Death 152

Signs of Approaching Death 153

Immediately after Death 154

Emergency Medical Services (EMS) 154

Removing the Body 156

Children 156

Suicide 157

Some Who Died at Home 159

Alice Clark 159

Jim DeMott 161

Lisa Knott 164

Elizabeth Krolick 165

Al Martin 168

Joyce Smith 170

Dorothy Stead 172

David Steiner 174

Herbert Wolf 175

John Wright 177

7. After Death 182

The Funeral 182

Grief 188

Practical Concerns 194

    Before Death 194

    After Death 195

    Settling Financial Matters 196

    Documents Needed 197

Conclusion: Living while Dying 198

Appendix A: Tasks and
Problems of Caregiving 201

General Care 202

    Appearance 202

    Hygiene 202

    Skin Care 203

    Sexuality 207

Health Care 208

    Nutrition 208

    Elimination 215

    Mobility and Falls 218

    Transfers 220

    Eye Care 222

    Sleep 222

    Cognitive Impairment 224

    Agitation 225

    Administering Medication 226

    Breathing Problems 230

    Oxygen 230

    Seizures 231

    Control of Pain 231

    Assessment 233

Appendix B: Additional Resources 238

General 238

Control of Pain 238

Living Wills 240

Caregiving at Home 240

Nursing Homes 241

Suicide 242
Grief 242

Appendix C: Pain Medications 245

Appendix D: Sample Letters 248

Appendix E: Caregiving and HIV 250
Introduction 250
Helping the Caregiver Cope 251
Infection Control Precautions for the Home Setting 254
Home Health Care Needs of Adults with HIV 256
Pain 257
Rights of HIV Infected Patients 258
End-of-Life Decisions 260

Appendix F: Michigan Dignified Death Act 262

Glossary 275
Bibliography 285
Index 289

Illustrations and Tables

Figures
1. Patient Log and Pill Schedule   96–97
2. Turning Someone from Her Back to Her Left Side   205
3. Finishing a Half Turn   206
4. Restraint System, Using Gauze Strips   220
5. Beginning to Transfer Someone from Bed to Wheelchair   221
6. Completing the Transfer   222
7. Preparing to Administer a Subcutaneous Injection   228
8. Administering an Intramuscular Injection in the Upper Arm   228
9. Preparing to Administer an Intramuscular Injection in the Hip or Buttock   228

Tables
1. Types of Support   114–15
2. Narcotic Analgesics for Severe Pain   245–47

Preface to the Revised Edition

Since the original publication of this book, much has changed in the care of the dying but more has remained the same. There are now more free-standing and in-patient hospices. And, more people are dying at home, in part due to increased awareness of hospice services and desire for a non-technological death, but also because managed care is forcing people out of the hospital into outpatient settings.

The pain and suffering of the dying has attracted considerable attention due to policy initiatives and to the assisted suicide movement, and there has been a major effort to educate physicians and nurses about improved pain treatment for the hospitalized dying. (The Project on Death in America, funded by the Soros Foundation, along with the Robert Wood Johnson Foundation is in large part responsible for raising scholarly, educational, and policy interest in the care of the dying.) Yet little progress has been made in improving treatment for the pain and discomfort associated with terminal disease. Although treatment in hospitals requires improvement, advances have been made in the technology, funding, and information about care for the dying at home. This new edition includes these advances.

The family and friends who care for the dying remain a little-understood group. Americans shy away from death, despite the current attention paid to it. Those family and friends who care for the dying experience their efforts as one of, if not *the,* most important accomplishment of their lives—their "finest hour." Diminishing the disjunction between people's sense of heroic accomplishment and the lack of a community to acknowledge their work is a goal of this new edition.

In the years since the book was first published, I have repeatedly heard from people who have used the book. Most use it as the originally intended guide to ongoing caregiving, but a significant number tell me they use it to create a community of shared experience, a context in which to evaluate and share their work. People end their care of the dying frequently judging it to have been the "best and worst time" of their lives, and yet they have no one with whom to share it. I have discovered that for many *Dying at Home* provides a silent community witnessing the caregiving experience. In addition to reading it in preparation for caregiving and during care of the dying person, caregivers read *Dying at Home* after their experience because it serves as a way to share what they went through and, by reading what others did and felt, to make sense of their own accomplishment.

After I finished the work that led to *Dying at Home*, I was asked to involve myself in an emerging problem in terminal care: care for those dying of AIDS. At first my involvement entailed applying the lessons learned from *Dying at Home* to improve care for a highly stigmatized group; eventually it led me to a systematic study of those dying of AIDS. Preliminary findings from that research inform the new section on AIDS care. The rather technical information included in that section fails to convey the crisis surrounding this care, especially as the epidemic moves primarily into minority communities where it competes with poverty and racism for primary attention in highly stressed, under-served, and disadvantaged groups. Dramatic advances in prevention and treatment outcomes experienced among whites have yet to be felt among minorities. Those dying of AIDS say it is easier to face death than the isolation and rejection they experience from having the disease. Their caregivers are often isolated and without traditional sources of support and sympathy. A key challenge in providing care for those dying of AIDS is to fight this stigma.

Driven by advances in medical technology combined with ever shortening hospitalizations, use of the home as the site of death will steadily increase. This will place significant demands on family and other informal caregivers. This responsibility goes far beyond the often exhausting and draining physical involvement demanded in care for the dying. It encompasses cultural work that involves assisting the dying person in living up to or enacting his cultural values, facilitating social contacts and resolving conflicts between the dying person and others, and assisting the dying person in creating a legacy. Caregivers are also acting in accord with their values: "This is how it is done in our family," they are saying as they model behavior for the next generation. As noted repeatedly throughout this book, caring for someone you love while he or she is dying can be one of the more intimate, meaningful, and loving aspects of a relationship; it can also be the most challenging. Most do not seek this; those who must do it say they would not have missed it for the world. Therein lies the dilemma and challenge for the caregiver of the dying: enabling the person you love to live out the last moments while preserving as much as possible of what you and the person value while facing the inevitable ending brought by the death.

Acknowledgments

There is a long and a short history to this book. Both are important to relate because they establish my reasons as well as my competence in undertaking this project. The immediate inspiration was my caring for a dying family member at home. My family was particularly fortunate and skilled in undertaking this responsibility; yet we found the task extremely challenging. My sisters, Suzanne Sankar and Pamela Sankar, urged me to use my training as a medical anthropologist and my expertise in home care to analyze our experiences for the benefit of others. Thus their suggestion marked the birth of this study.

Because my family was intimately involved with the origins of this work, they must be the first to be acknowledged. Leon and Renee Sankar were there to give us the support and guidance of the older generation. Suzanne and Pamela shared all of the caregiving, as well as critiquing the manuscript. Peter Cullinane and Gregg Gorton provided essential help as well as professional expertise. Frithjof Bergmann was my constant support and partner in caregiving and later encouraged me in the research and writing. Jandy Bergmann cared for the caregivers. Luke Bergmann contributed humor and warmth as well as the illustrations for the book. Sarah and Teddy Cullinane and Ariel Sankar-Bergmann were a constant source of joy for everyone. The serendipitous appearance of Jedd Sankar-Gorton was a blessing for all of us. Helen Waldron, George and Gaye Rosenwald, and Jane Barney were steady, constant friends and helpers.

The longer history of this work goes back to my graduate training, during which I was fortunate to learn ethnography from Roy Rappaport. Later, on a National Institute of Aging postdoctoral fellowship at the University of California–San Francisco Program in Medical Anthropology, I worked under the direction of Margaret

Clark. Through her I made contact with the University of California Home Care Program. For two years I worked as a member of the home care team, learning from the other members and studying them and the students and patients associated with the program. The team included me in all its deliberations and gave me open access to interactions with patients and students. All the members—the physician, nurse, social worker, pharmacist, and administrator—took it upon themselves to teach me their professional perspective on home care. They were good friends, valued colleagues, and wise teachers. I learned an immense amount from them. I wish to thank Steve Becker, Norma Criado, Joan Dunkel, Sato Hashizumi, Ron Finely, and Gary McCart. I also wish to thank the Division of General and Internal Medicine under the direction of Steven Schroeder for allowing the project to go forth. I was fortunate to have a final National Institute of Aging postdoctoral fellowship at the Institute of Gerontology at the University of Michigan, where I wrote up the home care research.

In the research and writing of this book I have benefited from the help and criticism of numerous colleagues and friends. Ingrid Deininger and Mary Lindquist taught me about hospice nursing. Cynthia Stewart, Steve Becker, Jerry Burns, and Francis Cornelius provided invaluable professional critiques. They are not responsible for the book's shortcomings, but they improved the final product immeasurably. Emily Abel, Nancy Hanke, Anna Holmberg, and Jessica Muller read all or portions of the manuscript and made valuable comments. My editors for the Johns Hopkins University Press, Anders Richter, Jacqueline Wehmueller, and Irma Garlick, improved the manuscript immensely and offered me constant reassurance and encouragement. Joann Cox at the Word Processing Center at Wayne State University typed several versions of the manuscript. The Wednesday night soup group supplied sustenance and companionship.

This has been a very difficult and painful book to write. To all the informants, who gave of their time and memories and who suffered from the recollection of their own pain, I owe my deepest thanks. Without them there would have been no book. I only hope that I have done their stories justice and that these case studies can serve as the kind of memorial the informants hoped they would be.

Some Who Died at Home

Alice Clark was fifty-six when she died of ovarian cancer. She had been a popular professor of sociology at a small college and was very involved in local politics. When she became so debilitated from the cancer that she could no longer work, she was cared for at home by her husband, Stan, and her three daughters. Her wide circle of friends helped with her care, as did her sisters. She wore a portable morphine pump for pain control and was moving about and functional until a few days before she died.

Jim DeMott, a corporation comptroller, was fifty when he died from brain cancer. His wife, Lucille, organized the care he received and provided much of it herself, which inflicted considerable physical strain on her. After he died, she had to be hospitalized on several occasions as she tried to recuperate from the strain of caring for him. They had just moved to assume new jobs. They had a new baby and a seven-year-old. Although Lucille did not know many people in the area, she was able to organize a network of people and agencies to help care for Jim. Jim's two adult children by a former marriage also came to help. Tensions over the division of his estate exacerbated hostility the older children felt toward Lucille. This created a difficult and sometimes discordant context in which Jim was cared for as he was dying.

Lisa Knott was only three years old when she died from leukemia. Her parents, Pat and Don, had noticed that their normally active and vivacious child was unusually quiet and sleepy. In addition, she had a strange sore throat and bumps on her neck. When the physicians finally diagnosed the leukemia, Lisa's white blood count was dangerously low. The hospital physicians elected to have a catheter placed in her chest to make the administering of the chemotherapy easier. There was a problem with the anesthesia during surgery to implant the catheter, and Lisa never regained consciousness. Pat and Don took Lisa home after two weeks when it seemed unlikely that she would emerge from the coma. Pat dropped out of school and Don was transferred to an office closer to home to help Pat with Lisa's care. During the three months they cared for Lisa, they received a great deal of social support from the church, the mothers' group Pat was a member of, and Don's colleagues. Lisa suffered from diarrhea. Even though she was in a coma, she also suffered from nausea and from pain in the week before she died.

Elizabeth Krolick was sixty-nine when she died from breast cancer. She had been a writer. After a long illness, her cancer metastasized rapidly and she had to be hospitalized while on vacation. She quickly became paralyzed and lost most of her hearing and eyesight. She was flown back to her hometown in an ambulance jet and admitted to the hospital there. She was discharged to her daughter Anna's home, where she lived another month and suffered from cognitive impairment and agitation from the brain metastases. Anna, with her husband, and her sister and brother—who both lived out of town—along with their spouses cared for Elizabeth. Her sister and brother took turns flying in to help Anna and her husband meet Elizabeth's intensive around-the-clock needs. Elizabeth's and Anna's friends also helped, and the family hired professional help.

Anthony Lane was a master plumber when he died at thirty-one of lung cancer. He was cared for by his companion, Laura Sweet. They had just moved to the Midwest from the South. Anthony's parents lived about an hour and a half away, as did his three children by his former wife, but the overwhelming burden of care fell to Laura. Anthony was in extreme pain and unable to work for eighteen months before he died. Laura worked only half time and stayed home to care for him. For almost one year they tried to pursue alternative therapies and went to a special hospital to receive chemotherapy supplemented by vitamin therapy. They altered their diet, which required much effort from Laura. Although Anthony was in extreme pain, he did not qualify under his health insurance for home care. Because they were new in the area, they had few friends or acquaintances who could help out. Laura provided almost all his care. The week before Anthony died, he and Laura moved to Anthony's parents' home. Then his parents helped to care for him.

Al Martin, an engineer, was fifty-five when he died from ALS (amyotrophic lateral sclerosis, or Lou Gehrig's disease). In the three years after he was diagnosed, he deteriorated quickly. He became completely paralyzed, suffered vision problems, and became unable to swallow. Worst from the perspective of his wife, Florence, was the complete personality change he underwent. From a kind and gentle man, he became abusive and extremely aggressive verbally, so much so that Florence was unable to find people who were willing to help her. Finally she located a woman with experience in caring for ALS patients, who helped three days a week. The burden of caregiving was intense and made worse by his abusive behavior to Florence and her teenage daughter by her first marriage. Al denied he was dying until a few days before the end.

Lawrence Quinn, a retired physician, was eighty-three when he died from lung cancer. During his retirement he had assumed full-time care for his wife, who suffered from a serious progressive mental illness. He was diagnosed and underwent an operation to retard the tumor growth. When he was discharged, his three daughters, two of whom lived in town and one in another state, hired several health aides to provide continuous care. His wife's condition deteriorated without his constant care, and she had to be institutionalized. The three daughters coordinated their efforts, each one assuming a different role in caregiving. After a brief hospitalization to rehydrate him, Lawrence died at home with his daughters nearby.

Carl Roehm was seventy-nine when he died from Alzheimer's disease. He was a former high school teacher. His wife, Mary, and his daughter Martha, who was a nurse, cared for him. Other children and grandchildren helped. Because Mary was unable physically to care for him and Martha worked, the family hired helpers, non-agency workers, whom they themselves trained to provide the continual care Carl required.

Joyce Smith was forty-five when she died from AIDS (acquired immune deficiency syndrome). She had managed a small business. She was cared for by her lover, Lucinda Klein. The diagnosis was made during a hospitalization for pneumonia, and she received extremely poor care and suffered serious discrimination because she had AIDS. Once home, she was too debilitated to work, and she required continual care for a decubitus ulcer and for the adverse effects of an improperly administered drug therapy that she received in the hospital. Lucinda and Joyce were assigned a daily nurse. Their apartment was small and cramped and it was difficult for Joyce to be comfortable. Because she had contracted AIDS from her former addiction to heroin, she didn't want anyone to know of her illness. Other than the nurse, Lucinda had little help in caring for Joyce, although she received emotional support from an AIDS support group. Joyce became more and more depressed about the disease and her impending death, and she committed suicide.

Dorothy Stead was seventy-one when she died from lung cancer. She had been a housewife all her adult life. Her husband, Joe, a retired carpenter, cared for her with the help of their daughter, who lived nearby. Dorothy was in and out of the hospital for several months after she was diagnosed. Finally, Joe brought her home, but no one at the hospital ever clearly told him that Dorothy was dying. For several weeks he tried to encourage her to eat and took her on outings to try to interest her in life. Her inability to eat and gradual mental deterioration alarmed Joe, and he sought help from a home care agency. People at the agency informed him of the terminal diagnosis and helped him care for Dorothy during the last weeks of her life.

David Steiner was eight months old when he died from a heart tumor. He was diagnosed after his mother, Bonnie, noticed that he seemed extremely listless. He wanted to sleep all the time, but when she put him down he screamed. While the diagnosis was being made, he was hospitalized, and Bonnie stayed in the hospital with him continuously. She and Jack, David's father, were able to take him home on a pass for several days. When he was finally discharged, they were told he might not live three months. The hospital encouraged them to bring him back when he appeared to be dying, saying that Bonnie and Jack probably couldn't stand to watch their young son suffer. David died that night in Bonnie's arms.

Herbert Wolf was seventy-one when he died from liver cancer. He had been a commercial artist. When his wife died, he had moved to live with his daughter Helena and had become active in the civic affairs of the town where she lived. He was also devoted to his two grandchildren, aged four and six, and spent considerable time with them. Herbert lived slightly more than three weeks after he was diagnosed; he had been very sick for the previous month. Helena took an emergency leave from her job as a social worker. Herbert didn't want people to know he was sick, and he refused to see his sons, from whom he had been estranged for several years. Thus Helena and her husband, Philip, received little support from friends and family and inadequate professional support. Philip assumed responsibility for running the house and caring for the children, and Helena cared for Herbert. Herbert became increasingly uncomfortable and agitated, and Helena finally suggested he go to a hospital so he would be more comfortable. She had expected him to return home, but three days after he was admitted, he died.

John Wright was seventy-two when he died from liver cancer. He and Helen, his wife, were co-ministers in their church. They counseled many parishioners and were the center of a wide circle of friends. As a young man, John had had testicular cancer from which physicians had predicted he would die. After his recovery he soon resigned from a distinguished professional career to devote himself to the ministry with his wife. When he again became sick, this time with liver cancer, he explored many alternative forms of therapy, including "spiritual surgery." Helen provided all his care except during his brief hospitalizations. Their three sons and daughter lived out of town but visited frequently. John did not experience pain and was able to do some work until a few days before he died.

Dying at Home

Introduction

Home Death: A Return to Tradition

"We did it!" exclaimed one woman after her husband died at home. Despite the tragedy and grief, a home death is a major accomplishment. With only one exception, the people in this book said this was one of the most—if not *the* most—significant accomplishments of their lives. A home death is intense, intimate, stressful, and excruciatingly exhausting. Yet more and more people are choosing to die at home, and their families* are choosing to care for them there.

Part of what is involved in the decision to care for a dying person at home is the desire to allow that person to live out life in as "normal" a way as possible. As several people expressed it, a home death allows the person to have the experience of "living while dying." This means treating the patient as an intact individual no matter how debilitated and fragile he or she has become.

People can submit to the indignities of being a patient when they know it is for a good reason—the restoration of health. They allow themselves to be scantily clothed in the presence of strangers, to have their modesty violated, to endure pain and discomfort, and sometimes to be treated like children by those providing care. Assaults on one's dignity seem like a small price to pay for health. But when health is irrevocably lost, when what little health one has is quickly seeping away, then what is left of life and personhood becomes all the more important. Then, too, physicians no longer have privileged knowledge about what is best for the person. When doctors can no longer hold out the promise of a cure or restoration of health, the goal of care must acknowledge and respect the dying

---

* *Family* here will mean a group of people who perceive themselves as having an enduring commitment and set of mutual obligations to one another. In this book, the term does not necessarily imply a blood or legal relationship.

1

person's values, moral history, sense of self, and autonomy. The maintenance of autonomy—that is, the recognition of one's humanity—and, importantly, the recognition that one is still among the living—becomes essential.

The **caregiver*** cannot stop the patient from dying but can help preserve the person's autonomy and stop others from treating him or her as no longer living. The caregiver can insist that the person be treated as an autonomous individual, with the rights and personal boundaries this implies. Achieving this goal in a hospital setting is especially challenging; there the basic rhythm of life is set by the institutional goals and necessary routines of diagnosis, treatment, and cure. The dying person does not fit into this context.

The Term *Caregiver*

Caregiver is the term frequently used in research to refer to the person with primary responsibility for someone whose disability or incompetence makes him or her dependent on another to accomplish the tasks of daily living. The dependency can be slight, requiring little help, or total, requiring around-the-clock supervision and care. *Caregiver* is used to signify the type of exchange involved. It specifically does not assume any particular emotional or social relationship between the two parties. Although, in the majority of home care cases, the person giving and the person receiving care are related, this is by no means always the case. Even when people are related, the nature of the tie may not provide much information about the caregiving relationship. For example, a distant niece or cousin or a divorced former daughter-in-law may become a caregiver. A friend, neighbor, or former lover can fill the role. It is the exchange between the people involved, not formal ties and obligations, which determines the caregiving role.

There are two important arguments against the use of the term *caregiver*. First, it fails to account for the case of multiple caregivers. Often several people will share the responsibility. Although at any particular time one person will be the main caregiver, the responsibility can be rotated among several others. Even when one person remains the primary caregiver, others assume significant responsibility and play key roles. Although in the text I have adopted the

---

* Boldface type indicates the first use of a term that is defined in the glossary.

convention of talking about and to a single caregiver, this book is meant to address all those significantly taking part in the caregiving process.

Second, the word *give* implies a one-sided relationship, whereas *caregiving*, except when the patient is extremely demented or comatose, is a relationship in which both parties participate. The person receiving care is active in that care. For this reason the term *care partner*, used in AIDS work, is more accurate in describing the relationship. Despite these arguments, however, I have chosen to use *caregiver* because its widespread use will make it more accessible and identifiable to the majority of people using the book. Many people providing the care view their work as a kind of gift; this, too, helps make the term *giver* acceptable.

Factors Contributing to the Trend

For the last fifty years, the tradition of people dying at home was set aside as advances in medical and nursing science offered the possibility that death could be delayed or prevented if a patient received adequate care in a hospital. Recently, several movements and events have come together to encourage a renewal of the practice of home death. These are: the popular movement to control one's own health and participate in decisions about care, the **hospice** movement, a growing recognition of the limitations of medical science, improvements in home-based medical technology and pharmacology, and changes in insurance reimbursement for hospital stays.

The Desire for Control

Since the early 1970s, there has been a widespread movement in health care which has encouraged patients and their families to assume more control over their health and the care they receive. Patient participation in decision making, informed consent, the holistic health movement, the women's health movement, and home birth are all examples of this move toward less paternalistic medicine and greater patient and family control over health care. Home death, which represents the desire of the terminally ill patient and the caregiver to assume control over the dying process, has been influenced by this trend. (See "Practical Concerns," chapter 7, for more on this subject.)

The Hospice Movement

Hospice refers to a philosophy of care which advocates that dying people be allowed to live out the rest of their lives free of medical interventions designed to prolong life and free of pain. Hospice agencies in communities throughout the country offer this care. Primarily, hospice care is provided at home, although there are some in-patient facilities. The formal acknowledgment of hospice treatment through reimbursement by **Medicare** and private insurance companies came about in the early 1980s. This official recognition has made it easier for people to die at home by providing them with some financial and professional support, by setting standards to regulate the professional care they receive, and by educating physicians, nurses, and the public about the home death alternative.

The Limitations of Medical Science

The limitations of medical science are becoming clearer. Medicine's dramatic early successes in greatly reducing the number of deaths can be attributed largely to improvements in public health and advances in the ability to treat infectious diseases. In the future, it is unlikely that there will be equivalently dramatic breakthroughs in the cure of fatal illnesses. Instead, there will be a kind of fine-tuning as medicine improves its ability to delay the onset of chronic disease, to keep chronically ill people alive longer, and to enhance their quality of life. Some even argue that medical science has gone too far and that some versions of **high-tech medicine** amount to an unnatural prolongation of life. Numerous high-profile cases concerning terminating life-sustaining technology (sometimes called "**pulling the plug**") have served to increase the general awareness of the limitations of medicine for saving the life of a seriously chronically ill patient. The increasing public awareness of the poor quality of life of those whose life must be sustained by high technology has led more and more people to forego such invasive or **aggressive medical treatment** and to opt for **palliative care**, that is, care for pain and symptom relief, either in the hospital or at home.

Advances in Home-based Technology and Pharmacology

While more people are choosing to die at home, advances in home-based medical technology and pharmacology are enabling a return home for patients who in the past would have had to remain in the hospital to receive treatment. Especially important are improvements in the areas of pain control, oxygen therapy, **intravenous (IV)** treatments, nutritional supplements, and **chemotherapy**.

Change in Insurance Reimbursement

Whereas these four factors represent the forces that are "pulling" people toward home death, the **prospective payment system** instituted in 1984 by Medicare can be seen as a factor "pushing" in the same direction. This system places financial constraints on the physician's ability to keep someone in the hospital who is not receiving active treatment. Except for the hospitals that have inpatient hospices, a person defined as terminally ill must be receiving treatment for pain or symptom relief to remain in the hospital. An exception is the regulation that allows a home-based hospice program to admit a dying person under its care to a hospital for five days each month. There is some flexibility in the interpretation of this regulation. The admission may in some cases be extended.

Problems of Caregiving

There is a period before death, lasting as much as several months or as little as a week, when the body begins to break down. This is a distinct time in the course of a disease. Several problems characterize it: the extreme fragility of the dying person, the often intense intimacy of the caregiving process, the significant levels of responsibility the caregiver must assume, the physical and emotional stamina required of the caregiver because of the unremitting nature of the task, and the cost.

The Dying Person

The dying person is fragile. This may seem obvious, but because so few people have had any close experience with death, and fewer still with caring for a dying person in their own home, the extreme fragility often comes as a surprise to caregivers. Many imagine that dying is somehow a clearly defined, almost robust process. They have no idea of how very, very sick a terminally ill patient is. Dying is often a gradual process of steady decline. Even when it seems the person can decline no more and still remain alive, further losses are possible. As one caregiver said, "It was like watching a drop of water on a leaf evaporate."

The patient continues to live throughout the process, making death also a time of life. This is the greatest benefit of taking on the responsibility of home care for a dying person, but it also causes the most problems. Common actions and activities that people take for granted can become overwhelming problems and ordeals for patient and caregiver. Eating, sleeping, going outside, taking a pill, drinking a glass of water, elimination, taking a bath, and keeping the patient clean, turned, and free from **bedsores**—all represent major undertakings for both. Caregiving becomes helping the patient to live while in the process of dying. To do this successfully from the perspective of both patient and caregiver requires great attention to and inventiveness with the simplest tasks.

There are special problems that both face—problems that do not simply represent amplifications and extensions of the everyday but are unique to the dying process: anguish, anger, **agitation**, and fear on the dying person's part, and crises and conflict between the caregiver and other family members. These problems can of course occur in a hospital setting; but there they tend to be somewhat contained by the strange and formal setting, one over which the participants have little control. Such is not the case in the home. There the caregivers must deal directly with the problems and devise solutions as best they can.

Intimacy

A home death brings out not only the best but also the worst in a person. Someone who is dying does not waste time on social gestures unless they express some deeper emotion. The rawness of the emotions, both positive and negative, may be overwhelming in a relationship already marked by strong ambivalence. For those who feel comfortable mainly with polite social exchanges, caring for a dying patient at home or even visiting may not be a good choice. Unlike the hospital setting, the home offers very few barriers to help control the emotional interactions. There are few or no strangers around, and the setting belongs to or is deeply familiar to the patient. This is not a public space, and the conventions of public exchange often do not exist. Conversely, the very fact that a kind of truth exists is judged by those who have undergone the experience as one of its greatest rewards.

The Caregiver's Responsibility

There are several dimensions of responsibility, all of which will be discussed in more detail in subsequent chapters. At this point I wish to establish the scope of the responsibility. Decision making is the most extensive area of responsibility, followed by actual hands-on care. For many caregivers, the responsibility of hands-on care is mitigated by professional help in the home. The extent to which the caregiver assumes responsibility for decision making depends on the dying person's own abilities in this area. For some people, the ability to make decisions remains intact until their death; for others, **cognitive impairment** clearly impedes it. The difficult situations, which are the majority, are those in which the patient may be, and probably is, experiencing some degree of cognitive impairment either from metastases to the brain characteristic of various forms of cancer, from dementia produced by a disease such as AIDS or Alzheimer's disease, from drug **side effects** or interactions, from malnutrition, or from severe depression. Speaking on behalf of the dying person then becomes much more difficult because the caregiver not only has to interpret what the patient cannot say but also has to assess whether what *is* said is actually meant. This is an extremely difficult area of care in hospitals as well as at home. The difference with hospitals is that they often (but not always) have a means to assess accurately the nature of cognitive changes, and they may have a social worker who can help interpret the person's wishes to other family members. In both cases, the caregiver's intimate knowledge of the person will be invaluable in most accurately interpreting his or her wishes.

Decision making simply refers to the countless small and large decisions one must make in the process of managing one's life and the lives of dependent family members. In this case, however, there are the added decisions necessitated by the care of an acutely ill person and all of the social, emotional, and material concerns that accompany the dying process. The range of decisions is quite large. There are those associated with ongoing life which must be dealt with despite the compelling nature of the situation. More specific to the caregiving context is the need to decide about social support—how it should be organized and what it should do; to adjudicate among competing claims for access to and control over the dying person; to assess the quality of care being received; to introduce or stop specific kinds of medical and nursing care; and to determine the nature of changes in the dying person's condition and assess ongoing problems such as pain management. I use this last form of decision making to illustrate how complex and challenging the responsibility can be.

When the patient leaves the hospital, the physician and nurses will assure the caregiver that palliative treatment will be available, meaning that treatment to alleviate pain and keep the person comfortable will be given. Although it may sound straightforward, drawing the distinction between life-prolonging treatment and symptom relief and pain control may be very problematic in reality. It now becomes difficult to distinguish whether a problem is caused by the disease process or by the dying process.

When one assumes the care of a dying person, these issues become crucial because physical changes or problems associated with the disease, or with other pathological processes, may be treatable or reversible, and therefore one might be able to increase the patient's comfort. For instance, extreme agitation may be due to **constipation** or an **adverse drug reaction**; both can and should be treated. Loss of appetite and sleeplessness, however, may be part of the dying process and not require treatment. Trying to distinguish is one of the most difficult, time-consuming, and continuous tasks for a caregiver. Clearly, if the person is not at the point of death, one would act. However, it is often not possible to predict when death will occur; in six of the cases reported here, for example, the patient was on the point of death either a number of times or for a sustained time, in one case for two weeks. In such cases decisions simply have to be made, and the caregiver must be able to do this or appoint someone else who is competent to do it.

Professional help should be available to those making such decisions. Unfortunately, however, the doctor and nurse may not be able to determine the cause of the problem without taking the patient into the hospital for tests, a decision that must be carefully considered. The caregiver with privileged access to the details of the person's daily condition may be the best judge of the cause of a change in a condition. This level of responsibility is a significant and singular aspect of the home care of the terminally ill. People who choose to monitor carefully and become involved in the hospital care of a patient may also assume such responsibility. Such a choice, however, also requires the ability to collaborate with and perhaps even to confront the hospital establishment, an undertaking that few may be prepared to accept, especially when someone they love is dying.

Ideally, the dying person should be involved as fully as possible in the decisions. Several factors tend to prevent this, however: the patient's cognitive impairment, the caregiver's desire to spare the dying person worry and needless hassles, and, frequently, the patient's desire to withdraw from the day-to-day and concentrate on taking leave of life. As the dying process accelerates, the caregiver assumes more and more responsibility for decisions, in many cases even having to speak for the dying person and interpret wishes concerning visiting, topics of conversation, and activities. Although the move home represents an attempt to maintain and respect the dying person's autonomy, the caregiver's need to speak for the patient on occasion can erode that autonomy. To preserve autonomy whenever possible, negotiate with the dying person beforehand about when and how the caregiver may speak for her or him.

The caregiver will need help in these decisions. Other family members and those intimately involved with the dying person may, in fact, insist on participating. Who participates besides the caregiver and dying person and how control and power are shared are potentially divisive problems that will be discussed in detail in chapters 3 and 4. An ideal model, briefly stated, is that any family member or intimate participating in actual hands-on care should be included in the decision making—if only for the valuable insight into the person's condition they might provide. In addition, those family members and intimates who are not able to be present but who wish to remain involved should be contacted frequently, at least once a day, more often if necessary.

There arise, however, situations where it is not possible to share decision making, for example, an emergency in which the decision to rehospitalize the dying person must be made immediately. Here the caregiver, along with the professionals, must act. Emergency situations and crises can easily occur with an acutely ill person. In order to prepare for them, the caregiver can ask the physician about possible crises and then discuss them with the patient, if possible, and others who participate in decision making. Preparatory discussions cannot anticipate all crises, as in the case of an IV that falls out, requiring a decision about reinserting it. The caregiver and others relevant to the decision-making process must accept that there may be times when the caregiver will have to act alone.

One must consider the needs of the living as well as those of the dying. Decisions made at a time like this are likely to affect the caregiver's future relationships to the people involved. Some situations are extremely difficult to handle.

Physical and Emotional Stamina

Caring for a dying person requires great emotional and physical stamina. Most people interviewed for this book said it was the single most exhausting experience of their whole lives. Many dying people have great trouble sleeping—from the physical pain, from mental anguish and fear, or from the disease process. Unfortunately, drugs often do not provide adequate sedation. They may, in fact, have the opposite effect. In addition, many dying people do not want to sleep: they say they don't need to because they have so little time left; or they're afraid that if they go to sleep, they won't wake up. Or, treatments may be necessary throughout the night. Quality night-time help is often the most difficult to obtain, and as a result, sleep deprivation over a long period is one of the most serious problems for caregivers. In some cases it leads to rehospitalization of the patient simply so that the caregiver can get some sleep.

When someone is dying at home, there is little relief for the caregiver. Home is the place people go in order to escape from the worries and frustrations of life. When someone is dying there, the home becomes the center of those worries and frustrations. One can leave home for breaks, for errands, and for work, but the patient and the need for care will always be there when one returns. The other side of the coin is that the dying person's presence at home, for many families, means that family life can go on, albeit in a constrained fashion—say, in the sickroom. In some cases a semblance of normality is maintained up until the patient dies. The ability to continue to live with the person while he or she dies is, for many people, an adequate trade-off for the inability to escape from the tension and pain of the dying process.

Expenses

Providing home care for a dying patient costs money. Insurance policies mainly cover skilled care and have minimal provision for a **home health aide**. The aide is what is needed most. The home health aide is someone who sits with the dying person and is competent at simple tasks like changing linen, cleaning up, and washing and feeding the patient. The caregiver may choose to provide all these services alone, but as the patient becomes more disabled, more than one caregiver will be needed. Family and friends are often extremely valuable in providing this supplemental help, but they must often miss work and lose money in order to do so. The hospice benefit in Medicare and private insurance is often not adequate to cover all the necessary care.

Deciding Whether to Become a Caregiver

Deciding to care for a dying person at home represents a commitment to quality care and to preserving the person's ability to live out the remainder of life with dignity. This commitment can also be made by caregivers who choose to have the person remain in the hospital. For a patient who is still hospitalized, the caregiver can act on this commitment by ensuring good care and the maintenance of personal dignity. The strategies described in this book will be appropriate for all caregivers—and for anyone who wishes to help care for an acutely ill hospitalized person.

For most of the people described in this book, there was no decision to make regarding care for the patient at home; they simply could not have conceived of another approach. But for others, the decision was not obvious, and some chose not to do it, or did not have to make the decision, because the patient died before discharge was possible. Those for whom this *was* a decision (and a difficult one) tended to focus on concerns that turned out to be inconsequential. Probably the single biggest concern expressed was the prospect of providing **perineal care** (care of the genitals) and coping with **incontinence** (spontaneous elimination of urine or feces). Not only was this of concern for people who were contemplating providing care but it was also one of the most frequent concerns expressed by those who sought to offer support to the caregivers. One informant responded to queries about how she could clean up her dying father's episodes of incontinence this way:

> You discover—at least for me—you discover that loving someone is such an overpowering emotion that it almost wipes out your repulsion about anything that is happening to someone else. You know once you have had a kid, if you really love your children, it would not cross your mind not to step in front of a bus instead of your child; you would just

do it. It is not even an issue. It is so obvious that it stops becoming an issue. And in the same way you don't say "Oh, yuk, I couldn't do that." People said, "How can you do this?" And I said, "How can I not?" You have to go; as long as you care for him, he is alive.

The other issue that was of great concern to people who had difficulty in making this decision was fear—the fear of having someone die in their home. Informants expressed fears that something supernatural would occur after the death, or more mundanely, that bad memories would keep them from using the room where death had occurred. Dying, like birth, is a stressful and intense but entirely natural process. There were no examples of "cold air" or "blue lights" after a death. The association of memories with the place of death is a fact. But these memories were positive as well as negative. People who changed residences after the death did so for practical reasons, not to remove themselves from the memory.

In some cases, caregivers confronted the possibility that the dying person would commit suicide, which tended to emerge during the course of care as the patient became more despondent. It was not an issue during the final period of life or during **active dying**, which is the focus of this book. I will discuss suicide, however, because it was of such concern to several informants and because, in the one case in which the patient did take her own life, it was done so traumatically that the caregiver remained affected by it.

Helena Wolf, who cared for her dying father, summed up her experience this way:

> People always talk about being pregnant and having children and this merging of body and emotions. But for me, since those were always positive experiences with happy outcomes, I was probably never stretched to the emotional extent that having to cope with [what] watching yourself lose something that you care about does to you. I mean, you know what the end is going to be. I knew he was never going to get up from that bed, and I think you protect yourself from that in two ways: you either stay away or you involve yourself because, as I always said, as long as he was there, he wasn't dead. That to me was the most important thing.
>
> It is not for everybody. I guess that is the other thing, it has to grow out of, you know, the nature of the relationship. I don't think it is the kind of thing you can do out of some sense of duty because it is just too excruciating to watch, and I don't think it is the kind of responsibility

that all children owe to their parents or [that] spouses owe to each other. All people are not capable of doing this. It takes a Herculean amount of strength that you are totally unaware of when it's happening that you have. It was only afterwards that I was aware of how drained by it I was. I couldn't not have done it and I don't regret it for a moment. It's made me able to sit here with you and to go and sit with our friend this fall and watch his wife die and understand how excruciating it was and not be afraid of that.

The Research for This Book

The Method

This book is an ethnographic account of the process of helping someone die at home. The data were collected through open-ended interviews with the caregivers of the thirteen people profiled in the previous section of this book. I did not set out with a preconceived model of how home death occurred, nor did I have a questionnaire or list of questions for the caregivers. I began the interviews by asking the caregivers to describe to me their experience of caring for a dying person at home. I asked them to be as detailed as possible and to include both positive and negative aspects. If the information was not presented spontaneously, I asked them to tell me about the role others played in helping provide care. I turned on the tape recorder and let the person talk. Everyone began with a detailed account of the terminal illness, which lasted anywhere from forty-five minutes to an hour and a half. Often the caregiver went on to talk in detail about the various aspects of the care that had been particularly positive or upsetting. If this was not volunteered, I would ask for it. In many cases I returned several times to talk with the caregiver, with the result that I have an average of five hours of interview data from each caregiver.

There was general agreement among caregivers as to which issues were positive and which negative. The issues on which there was broad agreement form the basis for the fundamental structure of this book. After the in-depth interviews had been completed, I continued to collect data on specific issues, to fill out and deepen my understanding of them, by talking with twenty additional caregivers and seven supporters. These were brief and specific interviews.

All the interviews were transcribed verbatim. I then analyzed the content of the transcripts into themes and selected quotations that illustrated the points being made. The appropriate selections were then returned to each informant to enable the caregiver to ensure the statements' accuracy and to remove any identifying details. Some informants made only minor changes; others added clauses or sentences to clarify their original intent. Most changed the grammar of the quotations to conform to the style of correct written prose.

The aim of this book is to present the actual experience of the caregivers. The account is organized around the issues or problems that the interviews indicated were most significant. I hope, in this way, both to provide an accurate picture of various forms of home death and to present information organized in a fashion useful to those considering or in the process of a home death.

This is not meant to be a study that defines the essential nature or processes of home death. To accomplish that, I would have needed a larger, and a racially and ethnically representative, sample. Although the sample represents a range of socioeconomic backgrounds, it is Euro-American. In my small sample of only sixteen (three of the informants are not specifically represented in the book because their cases duplicated others), one or two African-American or Hispanic informants could have been misconstrued to represent the experience of African-Americans or Hispanics with home death. Rather than run that risk, I confined the sample to one group. From the research I conducted with professional caregivers, hospital social workers, **discharge planners**, and people in hospices and **home care agencies**, I suspect that future research with other racial groups will identify similarities in the process of caregiving but significant differences in social support practices. Given the basic nature of the dying process, much of the information here is appropriate in any setting.

The Informants

Informants in this book came from many sources. The majority were referrals from home care agencies. Some responded to an announcement in a grief bulletin. Others were referred from colleagues who learned of my effort. The informants live in communities across the United States and represent a wide range of socioeconomic backgrounds. People gave graciously and openly of their time and their memories. The conviction shared by all of them that such a book was sorely needed and would have been a help to them when they were providing care stimulated their generosity. For many, there was relief in talking about the details of what had been an excruciating time. As many noted, no one really wants to hear what actually went on. What was an extremely emotional and traumatic as well as dramatic experience was, for most people, hidden in the past. All the informants in various ways displayed real courage in undertaking the tasks they accepted, a courage that in our society receives little recognition. Those who have gone through it know what it is about; those who may someday go through it will, I hope, be helped by this book.

Every effort has been made to preserve the anonymity of the informants. Although the case studies are presented nearly verbatim, I have changed the details of informants' lives and experiences as well as their names to disguise their identities.

How to Read This Book

The caregivers in this book were chosen to represent different types of relationships and different types of caregiving problems. These are in no way an exhaustive representation of all the different kinds of relationships involved in caregiving. After reading through the biographies that precede this Introduction, the reader can select one person whose situation most closely approximates his or her own and follow that person through the book. This will make it more manageable for those who do not have the time or inclination to read the whole book. This format, however, is *not* meant to prescribe a particular kind of caregiving relationship or pattern of interaction. The case studies represent the experience of individual people which readers may choose to apply to their situation—or not.

The book presents a variety of real-life solutions for the various issues and problems of caregiving. Some of the solutions were not successful, and some of these have been included, too. The quotations of caregivers who had a particularly significant or representative experience were chosen to illustrate each topic. Thus, not all caregivers appear in every section. It may be necessary to read the quotations of other caregivers in a particular section to find an illustration of a particular problem.

Not all caregivers, obviously, are representative of a category. For instance, Lucinda Klein and Joyce Smith were clearly not the typical couple who must face AIDS. Initially I had intended to write a separate chapter on AIDS. I decided not to in part because of the excellent material already available or soon to be available on the subject and in part because many of the processes and problems of active dying transcend disease boundaries. I kept this case study in the book as an illustration specifically of suicide and generally of the special problems same-sex couples have in dealing with the health care system and with families.

Name	Dying Person	Caregiver
Clark	wife	husband
DeMott	husband	wife
Knott	daughter (child)	mother
Krolick	mother	daughter
Lane/Sweet	man	woman companion
Martin	husband	wife
Quinn	father	daughter
Roehm	husband	wife
Smith/Klein	woman	woman companion
Stead	wife	husband
Steiner	infant son	mother
Wolf	father	daughter
Wright	husband	wife

Sitting with the dying used to be something people knew how to do. Tending to their needs, comforting their body and soul was a part of life, something children learned growing up. The dying now in some ways are different—they tend to be sicker, both because they may be very old and because medical advances keep the sick alive longer. This book will, I hope, help those who wish to sit with a dying person and help the caregiver cope with the new problems as well as to face old fears.

CHAPTER ONE

Taking the Patient Home to Die

For those about to undertake the home care of a dying patient, the hospital phase of care can serve as a valuable learning experience in that it can prepare them for assuming the full responsibility for care at home. By participating in the hospital care, caregivers can become familiar with decision making and develop a working relationship with the patient's physician. For patients and caregivers who avoid a hospitalization before the onset of the terminal phase of an illness, the material discussed in this chapter will be of assistance in working with the medical establishment while care is provided at home.

Participating in Hospital Care

Hospitals are institutions that represent technical expertise and knowledge. In the hospital setting, care is provided by highly skilled professionals. The body of knowledge, the experience, and the skill of physicians and nurses is formidable. Their knowledge is, however, general. That is to say, in many cases, they do not have intimate knowledge of a particular patient. They must apply general medical principles and past experience to the diagnosis and treatment of the individual patient. Usually the caregiver—the very person who knows the patient intimately and thus can become an expert concerning the patient—does not have access to that professional expertise. Knowledge of the individual patient is particularly important in the care of the dying, when relief of pain and discomfort becomes equal to—indeed, may surpass—the goal of diagnosing and treating the underlying disease.

A caregiver who actively participates in the care of a hospitalized patient has far more opportunity to observe the patient's condition and response to different medications than the professionals involved in that care. These observations can provide valuable information for professionals in their attempts to relieve the patient's distress and maintain comfort. Caregivers also play an important role in ensuring that the physician's orders are both appropriate and accurately followed by the staff.

Although there are compelling reasons to do so, it may be difficult for caregivers to become actively involved in the hospital care at a time when they are also dealing with their own and the patient's emotional needs. Many may choose not to do so and instead trust that the care received is adequate. For those who have made the choice to care for the patient at home, direct participation during the hospital stay can later benefit the home phase of care; by gaining experience in decision making and advocacy, and by establishing direct communication with the physician who will oversee the patient's care from the hospital, the caregiver is preparing for home care. The significant advantage of this involvement is clearly the ability to contribute to the patient's well-being and dignity. Many caregivers expressed a sentiment similar to that of Lucille DeMott, who said, "When you can't save the patient's life, when no one can, at least you can make sure that they are well cared for and have dignity."

The experience of Lucille DeMott in the different hospitals where her husband was treated illustrates the various roles a caregiver can play in ensuring that the patient receives quality care, especially when the patient is traumatized and suffering some cognitive impairment (this is often true of terminally ill patients). The caregiver potentially can make a contribution in the areas discussed below.

The Appropriateness of Treatment

When someone is dying, there are many physical and psychological interactions as the body shuts down, so that determining the pathological as opposed to natural source of any particular change may be difficult. Clinical tests can often dispel the ambiguity, but at a certain point the patient, the family, and the physician become reluctant to pursue more interventions, especially those which cause discomfort. Thus physicians and nurses may not be able to formulate the best approach for a particular problem unless they can also take into account the detailed observations of the caregiver. These are very helpful to the professionals as they assess the patient's condition.

LUCILLE DeMOTT: If you choose to be an integral part of the patient care process, which I did by being there and sleeping in the room, you see so much that is going on that no one else sees. The doctor isn't there all the time, the nurse isn't there all the time; no one else is there all the time except you and the patient. So you are in a unique position to gather information and to figure out ways to do things.

It is important to monitor whether or not the ordered treatment is appropriate for the patient. For example, the physician writes orders and nurses are trained to fulfill completely the order, even though it may not always be appropriate. For instance, Jim could not swallow a pill, but he was given pills according to the physician's orders. It was fairly easy to get the orders changed to an injection or liquid or to a crumbled pill, but I had to demonstrate that I knew he was having trouble swallowing and not just refusing treatment. This is really a problem when the patient is unable to speak for himself.

Procedures

Most hospitalized patients have to endure numerous medical proce-dures, from blood drawing to X-rays to far more complicated inva-sions such as **suctioning**. The caregiver can learn how these are done and, through talking with the patient, discover what about a particular procedure may upset, frighten, or hurt the patient. In many cases, the caregiver can work with the technician conducting the procedure to make it less traumatic.

LUCILLE DeMOTT: Another area where I helped was the way in which procedures were carried out. Jim had to be suctioned, but there were many different ways to suction a patient. The way that most respiratory therapists used was to come in on schedule and jam the tube down his throat. He hated that technique. I learned, by asking different therapists, that quickly inserting the tube in the throat made it easier because it prevented the gag reflex, but there was another, more humane, way of doing it. The patient would cooperate by swallowing and relaxing, get-ting the tube through his nose and throat and into the lungs. Jim minded the first technique, not the procedure, so I took over the job of suctioning him.

Bedside Nursing

That hospitals are primarily geared toward recovery can be seen from the current government policy of publishing the death rates of hospitals as a way of allowing the public to choose the "best" hospital. Although hospitals are ranked or grouped according to the severity of the illnesses they treat—the greater the severity of cases, the higher the expected death rates—the implication is that hospitals with higher death rates are inferior. This linking of quality of care to death rates is understandable but will compound the forces that already steer the hospital toward helping patients recover and away from assisting them to die. Such factors as the physician's view that death is a personal failure, reimbursement rates that may penalize hospitals for providing terminal care, and staffing patterns whose organizing premise is that the patients cared for are gradually improving, all combine to discourage the hospital from providing terminal care.

Hospitals are not geared for the intensive, noninvasive nursing care required by dying patients. Except in the intensive care unit, nurses expect patients gradually to assume more and more responsibility for their own care. The work distribution among the nurses is predicated on this notion. Nursing staff try to accommodate the needs of the dying patient, but unless the hospital is set up to offer hospice care, those needs usually come second to the needs of those who are recovering. Caregivers who are actively involved in patient care can make an invaluable contribution to the patient's well-being and quality of life by providing some nursing care themselves and by insisting on the provision of care that they are unable to give and to which the patient is entitled.

LUCILLE DeMOTT: There is a lot of room for becoming actively involved in patient care if you choose to do so. I think the patient gets much better care if you do. Keeping an incontinent patient dry is one important area. There are several techniques for keeping the bed and patient dry. The standard way is to use plastic pads under the patient. These are very bad for the patient's skin but easy to use because they are disposable and allow quick bed changes. After watching Jim's skin get bad, I learned from one of the nurses that the best way to care for the skin is to keep cotton next to it and the plastic pad under the cotton. I found that if I explained to the nurses that this was how I wanted it done, they would usually help me even though it meant more work for them. If they wouldn't help me or didn't have the time, I did it myself.

You need to be very vigilant. Most hospitals have rules about how many times one person can try to find a vein to put an IV in. In the hospital we were used to, the rule was two times and then you had to find someone else to do it. When Jim was hospitalized in another state, the nurse poked and poked and poked him, trying to find a vein. Finally I said, "You can't do that anymore." In my case the rule had been twice, so it took me a while to realize that this hospital had no rule. This is the kind of situation in which you need to know you have a right to intervene on the patient's behalf.

In some hospitals it is easier to get good patient care than others, and with some nurses and physicians it is easier to get good patient care than from others. But you just have to be the patient advocate. Everyone I have ever talked to who has had a seriously ill patient in the hospital for a long time found that they had to seriously monitor medications because they don't always work out right. You also have to monitor feedings. For instance, sometimes someone would bring in the food tray and leave it there but Jim couldn't eat by himself and no one would arrive to help him. I would never ever again assume that you get good quality care in a hospital. I would always be an advocate for good quality care. There is just an enormous difference you can make.

Communicating with the Hospital Staff

Although nurses provide most of the care for the dying patient, only physicians can prescribe pain medications and can diagnose the source of certain care problems. The association of death with a sense of defeat may make some physicians reluctant to be actively involved in the care of a dying patient or hesitant to accept a new patient who is terminally ill. As the patient's advocate, the caregiver may need to confront a doctor on such problems as adequate pain medication and, if need be, seek out one who is more willing to supervise the care of a dying patient.

When talking with health care professionals, one should be sure to use the correct technical name for the patient's disease or condition. Professionals will be much more responsive if they think the person they are talking to understands what is going on.

In the hospital, especially in a teaching hospital, the physicians who will care for the patient usually will not include his or her private physician. The patient's own doctor will instead act as a consultant and a link between the family and the hospital staff. The caregiver will need to communicate directly with the hospital staff in addition to consulting with the private physician. To make this communication as effective as possible, one must understand the chain of command in a hospital, because the physician delivering bedside care will often not be the one who makes the actual decisions about that care.

Most hospitals today take part in the training of **medical students** and **interns**. Even hospitals that do not function as teaching hospitals often have students working there as part of their training and to supplement the regular staff. The lowest person in the medical hierarchy is the third- or fourth-year medical student, who often wears a short white coat, as distinct from the longer one worn by an MD. The student will take the patient's medical history and will stop and chat. Students cannot make decisions or deliver treatment unsupervised. Immediately above the student is the intern, or **house officer** I or **resident** I. Interns have graduated from medical school and are MDs but require an additional year of postgraduate work before they become licensed physicians. The interns are supervised by more advanced residents. They can perform simple procedures on their own but do not make key treatment decisions except in emergency situations when no higher-level physician is available. As residents progress through their training—the length of which varies by specialty—they become more competent and assume more responsibility for direct patient care. In their final year of residency, they begin performing the most difficult procedures, including complex surgery.

Residents are supervised by an **attending physician**, who is the person most people think of as their doctor: this is the person they see on office visits. If the care a patient receives in the hospital is unsatisfactory or needs to be changed, it is the attending physician who has the ultimate authority to make the needed changes. In some advanced teaching hospitals, there is an intermediate level between the resident and the attending physician, the **fellow**. The fellow is a physician who has completed residency training and has gone on for advanced postgraduate work. The fellow assumes responsibility for the residents and is under the supervision of the attending physician.

The **chief of service** is the head of a particular specialty and is above the attending physician. This is primarily an administrative position, and in most hospitals the chief of service does not have power over the attending physician in matters of direct patient care. If a caregiver is extremely dissatisfied with a patient's care, he or she can inform the hospital's medical director, the person with ultimate responsibility for all the practicing physicians.

In a teaching hospital, it is important to remember that the patient can refuse to be the subject of **medical rounds**. Medical rounds are the teaching procedure in which the attending physician, accompanied by students, visits each patient and delivers a small lecture or holds a discussion concerning the patient's status. Most attending physicians are sensitive to the patient's feelings and perform their role in the hall outside the patient's room; some may not be as sensitive. If they find it uncomfortable to have this done in the room, patients have a right to refuse entry to the students. They can also refuse to have an intern or medical student perform a procedure. It is rarely possible, however, to refuse treatment from a more advanced resident or fellow.

In the hospital, it is the nurses who care directly for the patient; they play a crucial role that often goes unrecognized and undervalued. Developing good rapport and communication with the nursing staff will help to ensure that the patient receives quality care. The nurses will appreciate an acknowledgment of their role, and the caregiver can work with them in solving problems concerning the patient's care and well-being. Here, the caregiver's observations may provide especially valuable information to the nurse trying to diagnose the nature of a care problem, such as bedsores that fail to heal or pain management. A good nurse will care for the patient regardless of the caregiver's input, but in the case of the dying patient, the extra attention and input of the caregiver can only enhance the quality of care the patient receives.

Many dying patients are limited in their ability to speak for themselves because of weakness and pain, or cognitive impairment from the disease process, or both. They need someone to interpret their needs, to speak on their behalf, and when necessary, to make decisions about their care.

LUCILLE DeMOTT: If you are going to take an active role, like I did, it is important to find a physician with whom you can work. I found this out in another hospital where the physician there did not want to code* Jim and wanted to withdraw all treatment despite my objections. I

---

* A "code" means a decision has been made to resuscitate a patient. A "no code" is a decision not to resuscitate.

knew Jim was dying but I thought that he didn't have to die yet. The only way I got treatment for him was by being there all the time and documenting his condition so that I could demand treatment. After Jim had had two grand mal seizures, I felt that one more **seizure** would finish him off. There is a medicine available to prevent that from happening but the doctor said it wasn't justified in his case.

I got one nurse to stay after her shift who recorded observations of his tremors every few seconds and gathered enough data to build a case to give him the medicine. We took this to the physician and he was forced to give Jim the drug. I was able to make the case for what I wanted because I had been there all the time. So the bottom line is: if you have a patient who can't really care for himself, and if you have the time to stay in the hospital with them, I would advise that.

One absolutely crucial area where caregivers can and must communicate with the physician is in the decision to tell the patient that he or she is dying. This is clearly a difficult and touchy problem. Some doctors believe that a clear, even blunt, statement of the patient's impending death is required. Others feel that an indirect discussion is adequate as long as the patient indicates understanding, by some means, of the prognosis. The extent to which a physician is obligated to dispel the patient's denial is an area of medical practice which is surrounded by controversy. The caregiver can play an active role here in helping the physician assess the patient's ability to accept the truth and select the form in which it can be delivered.

ANNA KROLICK: My mother never really admitted that she was dying. She didn't actually deny it, but it was part of her strength that she insisted on living as long as possible. Yet she really wanted to go home. The physicians were very uneasy with what they called her denial. We had to stop several medical students from going in and saying, "Look, you have only a week or two to live." We felt that she would signal us when she wanted to know more about her condition and we waited for her to give us a lead. One day my brother was with her and she started talking about her funeral and told him exactly what she wanted and that she had had a good life. We felt that that was an adequate acknowledgment. Her physician was relieved. He wanted to be straight with her but he didn't want to "hit her over the head with it." He felt this was an adequate indication that she understood what was happening.

In summary, the caregiver can improve the quality of care the patient receives in the hospital in these ways:

- Assess the appropriateness of treatment.
- Monitor procedures.
- Perform bedside nursing.
- Communicate with the hospital staff.

The Decision to Discharge the Patient

The decision to discharge the patient implies that nothing more can be done or that whatever can be done, can be done at home. This is clearly a difficult time, filled with conflicting emotions. On the one hand the patient and family are eager to leave the institutional setting of the hospital; on the other, to do so is an implicit acknowledgment that the patient will soon die. Once the decision is made to withdraw life-prolonging medical treatment, there are three possible choices for continued care: to remain in the hospital and receive palliative care, to be discharged to a **nursing home** or in-patient hospice, or to return home and receive care there.

In some cases the physician is reluctant to discharge the patient. This happened with two patients in this study, both children. The doctors urged the parents of both not to take them home, saying they would not be able to stand the pain and suffering their children might endure. Both sets of parents were determined to have their children at home and convinced the physicians that they understood the possible outcomes and were prepared to cope with them. Fortunately, neither child experienced the kind of death described by the concerned doctors. The parents of both Lisa Knott and David Steiner discussed with the physicians all the possibilities and demonstrated that they understood and were willing to accept or at least try to accept the potential trauma of helping their child through the pain of dying. This reassured the physicians that they were not acting irresponsibly in allowing the patient to go home.

In some cases the patient is reluctant to return home. There are common reasons for this: the belief that adequate care at home is not possible, the unwillingness of the patient to discontinue treatment and acknowledge that he or she is dying, and the fear of the burden that care will place on the caregiver.

Going home to die is a traumatic transition. The informants in this book recognized the ambivalent nature of the move, but without exception they all viewed it with relief and eagerly anticipated having the dying person once again at home in the family, especially because this was the last time the person would be with them.

Discharge Options

Although hospitals are under fiscal constraints to discharge patients no longer receiving active care as soon as possible, they usually try to accommodate the caregiver's need for time to plan for the dying patient's return. In some hospitals it is an option for the patient to remain and receive only palliative care, sometimes because the hospital has designated hospice beds, and sometimes because the physician can arrange this by listing a diagnosis, such as pain management, that justifies continued stay.

In leaving the hospital, the patient can go to either a nursing home or home. If the choice is a nursing home, the discharge planner at the hospital will help arrange placement. The caregiver's input in selecting a quality nursing home is important. (Information on selecting a nursing home can be obtained from a local **Area Agency on Aging** office or from the state **Ombudsman's Office for Aging Affairs**.) In some cases a **phased discharge** is possible: the patient goes first to a nursing home, to help stabilize the condition, and then returns home. This is the plan that Anna Krolick and her brother and sister had worked out:

> When my mother was hospitalized, the physicians told us she had six months at the outside to live. We had several problems to confront. She desperately wanted to walk again and had only recently become paralyzed. Also, we wanted to move her back home, which was seven hundred miles away, and she had to be strong enough to make that move. Finally, I was going to care for her and my sister and brother wanted to spare me the burden as long as possible.
>
> We hit upon the idea of having her go to a rehabilitation hospital for several weeks. She liked this idea because it would help her walk; and it would postpone the time when I would be assuming full care for her. Having this plan also helped us buy time in the hospital. She wasn't receiving treatment, and the hospital had started to push us to have her discharged. With this plan, they backed off. The problem was in getting her accepted to a rehab hospital because they don't like to take terminal patients. We got her accepted one place because her determination to

walk impressed the person who assessed her and because my sister knew someone on the admissions committee.

In planning the discharge caregivers must consider both their own abilities and the patient's status and desires. Depending on the patient's situation and the locale, there may be different options to select from in tailoring a plan of care to suit the caregiver's abilities and the patient's needs.

Planning the Discharge

Before the move home can take place, there are several things that must be attended to. Some are done in the hospital, such as learning simple nursing techniques, understanding the drug regimen, and planning the logistics of the move. Other problems must be solved outside the hospital, such as ordering medical equipment, deciding if additional help will be necessary and arranging for it, and selecting the room in the house where the patient will live. Chapter 2 deals extensively with the issues and problems involved in determining the kind and amount of professional help needed. The section that follows here describes the decisions that are made while the patient is still in the hospital.

Hospital-based Preparations

If the caregiver understands what preparing for home care entails, he or she will know what information must be obtained before the patient is discharged. Most hospitals will alert the caregiver to at least some of the preparations that must be made, and the caregiver needs to ask for information about the others. The preparations fall into three categories: medications, nursing procedures, and transfers. Transfers must be arranged both in the hospital and at home and are discussed on page 34.

Medications. Most patients are discharged from the hospital with several medications that they are to take at home. The caregiver needs to understand the purpose and importance of the different medications, and so should ask the physician to explain what each medication does and draw up a prioritized list. Then, if the patient begins to refuse medications or if swallowing becomes very difficult, the caregiver will know which medications have priority. In Anna Krolick's case this was particularly important:

After the initial crisis during the transfer home, Mother began to refuse to take her meds. This was also partly due to the mouth sores from her chemotherapy, so the nurse suggested we stop all medications. Within a day or two she became extremely agitated. Finally, my sister realized that the Decadron [the treatment for her brain tumor] was missing and we began giving it to her. No one had told me how crucial it was. Without the drug my mother would have died very quickly. My sister figured out that if we crushed it and placed it in Gatorade, which disguised its taste, we could get my mother to take it. This helped immediately, but she never recovered the mental status she had had before we discontinued the drug.

Lucille DeMott's experience was completely different:

I wanted to know how to help Jim die if that seemed to be the best decision. The physician simply answered that without Decadron he would become unconscious and die.

Neither of these patients had very long to live, but both wished to live as long as possible. In Mrs. Krolick's case, the nurse's erroneous advice about the medications and her daughter's lack of knowledge of them almost prevented this.

Information about medications must be obtained before the patient is discharged. For each kind of medication there are five areas in which information must be obtained:

1. Priority
2. Alternate forms
3. Scheduling
4. Purpose and administration
5. Changes

1. *Priority.* With a *prioritized list of medications* that also spells out their functions, the caregiver can avoid eliminating the patient's most important medications. (If an important drug *must* be eliminated, the caregiver will know the consequences beforehand and be prepared.) If the patient refuses medications, the caregiver can use extra effort to make certain that key medications are taken. The hospital physician may prioritize the medications for the caregiver; otherwise, a doctor working with the home care agency or hospice may help. At home, decisions about medications may have to be made under stressful circumstances. Thus, for medications as for

other areas of care, it is better to ask the questions while the patient is in the hospital and the responsibility for care lies with others.

2. *Alternate forms.* In many cases the patient will refuse medications not out of a wish to die but because swallowing is so difficult. (Appendix A discusses other ways to administer the medications when the dying person is unable to swallow.) Difficulty in swallowing can be the result of weakness or a side effect of chemotherapy, which can cause serious mouth sores. Most drugs have alternative forms; that is, they can be administered in pill, liquid, suppository, or injectable form. Find out which have alternative forms. If a medication is available in only one form, find out whether there is another medication that can be substituted for it.

3. *Scheduling.* Most medications must be administered every six, eight, or twelve hours. If the goal in home care is quality of life, it will be desirable to avoid waking the patient for a pill. Ask if the time periods are absolutely essential to the drug's effectiveness; they may not be. Also, a suppository or injection might be less disturbing to someone who is sleepy and might be considered if the schedule of dosages is very important, as it is for pain medications, for example.

4. *Purpose and administration.* Again, the best time to discuss with the physician the *purpose* of the medications and the *way they should be administered* is during the patient's hospitalization. It is often difficult to reach physicians by phone, and emergency room visits should be avoided (for reasons explained later). When a patient is dying, the doctor will usually take time to explain what the medications are for so they can be used responsibly.

5. *Changes.* Prior to discharge, *changes of medication* are sometimes made and the patient placed on new medications that are easier to administer at home. This is especially true of pain drugs. Make sure the professional staff has taken time to evaluate the effectiveness of the new medication. When the patient is not stabilized on a medication, it can create a difficult transition from the hospital to home if pain is not adequately controlled or if the patient has an adverse reaction to the medication.

Nursing Procedures. Caring for the terminally ill at home requires the performance of many nursing procedures. It is part of a nurse's job to provide patient and caregiver with instruction, but this generally includes only standard procedures such as transfers. In the hospital, it is possible for the caregiver to notice details of care and ask about those which seem particularly effective. Observing a skilled professional work is often the best way to learn. Even if someone is hired to do these procedures at home, it is a good idea for the caregiver to learn them. It is always possible that even the most reliable aide or nurse will not appear for work and that a replacement cannot be found in time, or that a crisis will arise when there is no plan to have help in the home. Even if the caregiver cannot perform the procedure, by knowing how it is done, he or she can instruct someone else, such as a neighbor or friend, who is helping out.

What the caregiver needs to know will depend on the individual patient's condition. Some of the more common procedures are: intermittent **catheterization** (inserting a tube into the patient's urethra so the bladder can empty); transferring the patient from bed to wheelchair, turning the patient so the bed can be changed; positioning (placing the patient so bedsores do not develop); the care of stiff limbs; eye care; mouth care; skin care; injections; **disimpaction** of bowels; administration of **enemas**; and other, more specialized procedures associated with different technologies. Training in all the procedures is available from a home care or hospice nurse. The cost of this training is reimbursed by insurance.

While helping to care for the patient in the hospital, one can learn what the patient is able to eat and how to encourage eating. This subject will be discussed in greater detail in appendix A, but for now, it is important to know that in the hospital the caregiver can request a conference with the dietician to learn of simple nutritious foods and tricks to encourage patients to eat. The American Cancer Society also provides literature containing recipes for patients who have trouble eating.

Before the patient leaves the hospital, nurses will usually supply the caregiver with some of the materials needed for home care. The caregiver can ask for more of certain supplies that have been particularly effective in the hospital. For instance, certain kinds of medical swabs are difficult to obtain in stores; a good initial supply of tiny plastic cups (for holding and administering medications) and long cotton swabs can be invaluable until a store that sells them is found.

Home-based Preparations

Medical Equipment. Most people who die at home become so frail that they require at least a hospital bed. Many require far more equipment. If the patient is being discharged from a hospital, the discharge planner will explain what kinds of equipment will be needed. The most frequently required equipment includes a fully electric hospital bed, which raises and lowers, allowing ease in turning the patient, changing the bed, and positioning the patient; a **commode**, which is a portable toilet allowing the patient to eliminate at bedside; a wheelchair; a **walker**, which is a four-legged device that makes walking easier for those well enough to stand on their own; and a lift, which can be used to help move a patient from the bed to the wheelchair. The patient's condition and abilities will determine what equipment is needed.

More technical equipment is sometimes needed. An **infusion pump** is used to maintain the patient on a high dose of medication by continuously injecting the medication through a **subcutaneous** (under the skin), intravenous (in a vein) or IV, or **intrathecal** (into the spinal canal) needle. Oxygen can be given continuously, and nutrients and chemotherapy can be administered through IVs in the home. Suctioning equipment is used to keep the patient's air passages free of mucus.

The **durable medical equipment (DME)** can be leased from medical equipment companies. Often the home care agency that cares for the patient has a preferred provider and will arrange the delivery of the kind of equipment needed. If there is no home care agency involved in the patient's care, the hospital discharge planner will have a list of the companies in the area, and the caregiver will need to call several and compare prices and service policies. Try to select a company with a good service record. Ask for a list of customers and call them to check on the company's performance record. Malfunctioning equipment can have serious consequences, including endangering life. To avoid some potential problems, have the company try out the equipment when it is delivered. It is easier to return it at this time than when the patient is already using it, which is what Anna Krolick learned:

> We had barely gotten my mother settled in bed when we tried to raise the bed and discovered that only the foot raised. The move had been so traumatic for her [that] we didn't want to take her out of bed again, and the idea of a strange repairman coming was more than anyone could take. We decided to just make do, but it was difficult. When she got a little better and we had her out in the wheelchair, the nurse played around with the bed and fixed it.

A portion of the rent for medical equipment is covered under most insurance policies. In some cases, home care agencies and hospices have their own equipment, usually because former patients and families have donated it, and they may loan it free of charge. Equipment such as a hospital bed can be purchased. This arrangement has a tax benefit because, after it is no longer needed, the bed can be donated to an agency. The donation is tax deductible.

Choice of Location. Deciding where in the house to settle the patient requires serious consideration because the location will affect the ease with which the patient is cared for and the caregivers' well-being. For some people there will be so little space, or the demands of care will be such, that the choice will be made for them. For others, several factors must be weighed before the most appropriate location can be chosen. Some are purely practical concerns.

Access to the outside and to the rest of the house is important. If the plan is to take the patient outside for a walk or to sit in the sun, or if the patient has to return to the hospital for any reason, easy access to the outside is desirable.

Nearness to the bathroom is essential for patients who can still walk. Being able to eliminate unaided and in a customary fashion is psychologically important to most people. It symbolizes one's continued control over one's body. In a terminal illness, so much is out of control that elimination becomes such a symbol and measure of physical deterioration. The patient should be assisted in maintaining this ability as long as possible. Selecting a room close to a bathroom will help prevent accidents, which the gradual loss of body control makes inevitable.

Included in the physical considerations should be attention to whether the room is sufficiently warm and well ventilated. As terminal illness progresses, it becomes more difficult for the person to keep warm. At the same time, ventilation may also be a key: depending on the illness, the body's productions can be foul smelling, and adequate ventilation obviously becomes necessary for both patient and caregiver. Ventilation is also particularly important for people suffering from AIDS, for many of them develop an extreme sensitivity to smells. Lack of adequate ventilation can make their lives especially difficult to bear.

Perhaps most important for the well-being of both the dying person and the caregiver is the effect that placement will have on social relationships. The degree of interaction between the patient and the caregiver and family will be affected by location of the sick person's bed. If the person is completely bedridden and requires considerable care, it is helpful if there is some space between the person's room and the caregiver's, so the caregiver can "get away," even within the same house. If the patient is alert and desires social contact, easy and comfortable access will be important. If the house is large enough, it helps for the dying person's area to be separated from the main social area. In this way guests and family can withdraw when the person is tired or does not want to see anyone. In this arrangement, the family can also maintain some privacy and separation from both the patient's visitors and the professionals involved in the person's care.

Of course, all of these concerns must be disregarded if the house is so small that there are no choices to be made, or if the patient expresses a strong desire to be in a particular room. Here are accounts of how different families chose a location for the patient, the problems they encountered, and the solutions they devised.

LUCINDA KLEIN: We were in a small apartment. Joyce's bed was in the living room. We had to get a hospital bed because she had to be propped up to eat. It was all crammed in there. It was really uncomfortable. We had a hospital bed and bedside commode and collapsible walker and a wheelchair. It was a walk-up apartment two flights up. It was really just a prison, which is what she called it. That made it terrible. I was making desperate attempts to find another apartment and couldn't find anything with more than one room that we could afford. It was very discouraging.

STAN CLARK: One of the things Alice had a horror of was a memory she had of visiting a dying friend and seeing him set up in the living room where his protective wife was able to control all the social interactions he had. She said the whole living room scene was a ghastly one. We put her in the den, which gave her some privacy because there were some doors we could close. In the end, the last week or so of her life we moved her upstairs. She should have been upstairs longer because we have an all-glass house and the sunsets are absolutely spectacular and were a great source of pleasure to her. I don't know why we didn't do this sooner.

HELENA WOLF: When we came back from the hospital, Father went to his room. We cared for him there and never really considered any other place. This was his bed, his room—this was clearly where he wanted to be. It made things hard for me, having to run back and forth all the time. But he wanted privacy and he was able to have it his way.

The Transfer Home

Once both the hospital- and home-based preparations have been made, the actual transfer of the patient can be planned.

The dying person is fragile and has limited physical and emotional reserves. The move home, even when it is well planned, can be extremely exhausting. The discharge planner at the hospital and the nurses caring for the patient can help with some of the planning and preparation, but their job is only to discharge the patient from the hospital in a safe manner. The caregiver will have to assume responsibility for situating the patient at home safely and comfortably with a minimum of trauma. The stories of three families will illustrate how strikingly different this move can be.

STAN CLARK: When Alice was ready to come home from the hospital, everyone was there in her room—everyone in the hospital that had ever had anything to do with her. Only one of my nieces had come to bring her a present and had picked it out herself and it was this colorful scarf. It was funny because Alice never wore anything on her head. I had come on home ahead of the ambulance, and some people stayed waiting there with her, my kids and everyone. The rental place had already set up the bed. Anyway, she came in on this stretcher coming out of the ambulance, leaning back like she was being toted around by some servants, making the homecoming a triumphant return from the wars. She had this scarf on and some other funny thing. The doctor was there within ten minutes and was concerned with all sorts of details of Alice's comfort and quality of life and doing things like picking up the puppy and putting it on the bed for her, making Alice feel like she wasn't dead yet.

LUCILLE DeMOTT: We had asked for an ambulance to take Jim home because this was a totally bedridden person and his room was to be on the second floor, which meant going up a narrow set of stairs. The hospital transport system had no **gurney** to get him up the stairs with. Finally two men grabbed him, one on each leg, and carried him into the house and up the stairs. He was mortified, I was mortified. It is real interesting how those insensitivities can drive you crazy at a time like this.

ANNA KROLICK: We had arranged the move well. I was at the hospital with my mother. My husband had waited at home that morning to receive the hospital bed. He had gone to my mother's apartment and brought over her Oriental rug, which she loved, for the floor of her room. We were all very nervous. My mother was especially anxious. I raced home and arrived just ahead of the ambulance. The transfer was easy. My mother was glad to be home. She said, "Now I feel I can really relax."

In the last-minute rush we hadn't gotten clear instructions on all the meds. That night we stopped most drugs and may have given her one drug incorrectly or she might have been so exhausted from transfer that she temporarily stopped breathing and we thought she had died. She recovered but was terrified by the experience and never slept at night again.

A smooth transfer is the culmination of good planning on everyone's part, but even a good plan can go wrong. Depending on the frailty of the patient, caregivers need to anticipate problems and build in as much flexibility as possible to allow themselves to cope with the problems. In this highly symbolic and emotionally charged process, even little problems have consequences that can seriously affect the well-being of all involved.

Rehospitalization

Once the person is home, circumstances may arise that cause the caregiver or dying person to consider a readmission, at least temporarily. If this happens, the rehospitalization must be well planned. But whatever the reasons for it and no matter the amount of forethought, readmission can prove difficult and exhausting for the terminally ill.

Reasons for Readmission

Respite
There are times when caregiving can become too physically and emotionally draining for the caregiver to continue. It is impossible

for a caregiver to function with the chronic and severe sleep deprivation that can accompany the care of a dying person. In many cases, other family members—and friends possibly—combined with formal support, can step in to allow the primary caregiver time to recuperate. Some form of **respite** is essential in prolonged caregiving. Under the Medicare hospice benefit, it is possible to admit a patient to the hospital for five days a month for caregiver respite, and other insurance plans may also have some such provision. If not, a sympathetic physician can often arrange admission. Caregivers in this situation should see the respite admission as a reasonable and appropriate action that will allow them to continue caregiving once they are rested.

> HELENA WOLF: Finally, by the end of the second weekend—and I don't know why weekends seemed to be the worst—he had become so uncomfortable and sore, and complained almost constantly of hurting here and there, and not sleeping. There didn't seem any way to get him any relief. It was getting very difficult for him to get up and go to the bathroom. Either we were going to have round-the-clock nursing or something was going to have to happen. I finally said, "Lookit, I think you are very uncomfortable and you should go somewhere, the hospital or a nursing home, someplace where you can get more careful care. This is not good for either of us." And he accepted that immediately. We thought somehow we could sort of get things under control, get things sorted out and then bring him home. I did not think that my father would be dead in four days.

Treatment of Reversible Conditions
Although the illness may clearly be terminal and the underlying pathological condition will soon result in death, acute, potentially reversible conditions can arise. The question then becomes whether to treat them or not. There are clear signs when death is near. These are usually different from acute, reversible conditions. Perhaps someone with two months or less to live suddenly runs a high fever. If the infection causing it is not treated, it will precipitate death. When the dying person is alert, functioning, and retains the desire to live, most people opt for short-term hospitalization. It is always possible that the acute condition cannot be reversed and that the patient's condition will worsen with or without hospitalization.

Again, it is important to discuss *before* the hospitalization the extent to which life-sustaining treatment should be used.

Relief of Pain and Other Symptoms

Sometimes the dying person becomes so uncomfortable from pain and other symptoms of disease that remaining at home is no longer possible if a good quality of life is to be maintained. In such cases a short-term admission to assess and treat the problem is possible. Often these planned admissions are extremely beneficial, and the patient can return home with a greater level of comfort and safety.

Change of Plan

In some circumstances, people who intended to have death occur at home find that this is not possible, and the death occurs elsewhere. Death can occur unexpectedly during a planned admission; it can also occur in the hospital as the result of a clearly made choice, such as one of the following:

Coma.   When the dying person slips into a **coma** and no further communication is possible, caregivers may decide that they have fulfilled their duty to the patient and can no longer continue the caregiving. The dying person may then be admitted to a hospital or, more likely, to a nursing home. The caregiver can visit regularly, but the physical strain of caregiving is relieved.

Comfort and Safety.   In the advanced stages of some diseases, the body deteriorates to such an extent that the patient cannot be safely and comfortably cared for without a level of skilled care impossible to deliver at home. Simply turning a patient who has advanced bone cancer, for example, can cause bones to break and inflict excruciating pain. In such cases the dying person's quality of life suffers so much that the rationale for a home death—namely, to enhance the quality of life—is undercut, and the hospital or nursing home becomes the only feasible alternative. When infectious wastes threaten the health of the caregiver and caregiving household (in the case of a person with AIDS, for example), hospitalization should be considered.

Impairment of the Caregiver.   In the course of caring for the dying person, the caregiver may become exhausted and worn down or may develop physical problems that make it impossible to continue. If the extent of problems and exhaustion cannot be alleviated by an admission for respite, it may require a permanent admission of the terminally ill patient to a hospital or nursing home. An in-patient hospice with unlimited duration may provide the ideal solution for the impaired caregiver and the dying person, but, unfortunately, there are still few of these in operation.

If the caregiver feels it is simply no longer possible to give care, it is possible to take the patient to the hospital emergency room. This can be done without support of the professionals involved in the person's care. Any one of the numerous conditions that afflict the dying (e.g., dehydration, sleeplessness, poor nutrition, pain, agitation, severe constipation) can be adequate to secure admission. In this situation, it is important to take patients to the hospital where they have a medical record that documents their code status (including whether **heroic measures** are to be used to prolong life). This precaution avoids the use of **life support systems** against their will, for example. The caregiver needs to accompany the person to the emergency room and point out to the staff there the indications in the patient's chart and his or her wishes concerning heroic measures.

The Wish of Patient or Caregiver. Sometimes the dying person does not want death to take place at home after all. Although having wished to be nursed at home, the patient may fear the effect that the death will have on the family or may wish to reduce the burden that caregiving is causing. Often counseling from hospice workers and the reassurance that a hospice worker will be present while the person is actually dying can reassure both the dying person and the family. When this reassurance is not sufficient or when the burden is too extreme, the patient's wish to receive institutional care should be respected.

The dying person who is not a hospice patient may not qualify for a hospital admission and may instead be sent to a nursing home. With a serious shortage of nursing home beds, admission is not automatic. Thus, if the dying person clearly wishes to avoid death at home, the home care agency involved needs to begin working on the admission early. If the death appears imminent and the person is a hospice patient, he or she should qualify for an in-patient hospice admission; however, if the death is not likely to occur soon, the patient may have to be admitted to a nursing home where the hospice people may continue to follow the progression of the illness (the willingness of hospice personnel to do this depends on the individual agency's policy).

Considering Readmission

There are several factors to be taken into account when considering hospital readmission of the terminally ill.

The Discomfort of Travel
The trip to the hospital for someone who is in pain or is greatly fatigued can be an excruciating experience even when the distances are short. Depending on the physical condition and degree of frailty of the dying person, the actual physical move may be more painful than the possible benefits to be derived there, and for the very frail the trip may actually be life-threatening.

> STAN CLARK: We had Alice readmitted twice for blood transfusions because that would make her feel better. The physician said that if she went to outpatient it would not be very comfortable because you can't just dump blood in—it takes several hours to transfuse. We arranged a time when the nurses who we had at home would be on the oncology floor and admitted her then. She went two times, and the last time she said she couldn't go again. It was never a therapeutic procedure for her but a question of comfort.* But getting her to the hospital was too difficult. It was a tough experience for her.

If the person you are caring for requires admittance through the emergency room, make sure there is a **durable power of attorney** in effect for him or her.

The Process of Readmission
Once at the hospital, the problems may increase. Few hospitals can admit a patient immediately to a bed even with prior arrangements. Hospices have direct admit privileges, which means they can admit a patient directly without going through the emergency room. Home care agencies do not have this privilege. They admit terminal patients through the emergency room. This can involve a long wait for the patient, lying on a gurney in an emergency room bay. With the best of preparations, this wait usually lasts a minimum of one hour, and if the emergency room is busy, it can last five or six hours. For a

---

* The blood transfusions made her more comfortable by increasing the red blood count, which gave her more energy.

fragile, fatigued patient who may be in pain, waiting on a hard gurney for several hours in the commotion of the emergency room can be a harrowing experience and can seriously harm not only the quality of life but also the little physical health he or she possesses.

Life Support Intervention

In any hospitalization for the terminally ill, a life-threatening situation could develop. For that reason it is imperative that consideration be given to the use of life support interventions such as **cardiopulmonary resuscitation (CPR), ventilators, antibiotics,** and intravenous nutrition and **intravenous hydration.** These decisions should be made before the patient is discharged home in the first place, and they should be assessed *before* a readmission. The family and dying person may wish to rule out the use of any life support intervention or only the most intrusive ones such as CPR or ventilation (sometimes intravenous antibiotic therapy is considered to be intrusive, as well).

If the patient and family have agreed that no heroic measures will be taken to prolong the patient's life (and this is usually the case with patients who choose to die at home), then readmission to the hospital runs the risk that the patient might be placed on life support systems, despite prior agreements, if a crisis develops during the admission. When the patient is admitted through the emergency room, the physician in charge, in all likelihood, will not be the patient's primary physician and may not know of agreements the patient and family have reached regarding life support. To avoid such a possibility, the patient's doctor should alert the emergency room personnel to the purpose of the admission and inform them of any agreements concerning the use of life support systems. If at all possible, it is the patient who should tell the emergency room staff and admitting physician of those decisions. If the patient is not able to do so, the caregiver must. As a further precaution, the caregiver or other responsible family member should accompany the patient at all times during this process and be prepared to contact the primary physician if any problems arise. To facilitate this process, inform the doctor, the office, or the answering service when the patient is actually on the way to the hospital.

For many people, caregiving for a home death begins in the hospital. When the assessment is made that the patient will soon die, a choice must be made whether the person will remain in the hospital and receive palliative care, go to a nursing home, or go home. In deciding to care for someone at home, the caregiver needs to assess carefully his or her strength, sources of support, and stamina, as well as the flexibility of the household where the dying person will live and its ability to cope with the strain. Helping someone die at home can be immensely satisfying, but it also requires considerable strength and stamina and must be carefully considered in order to ensure the welfare of all concerned.

CHAPTER TWO

Strangers in the Home: The Use of Formal Support

The Functions of Formal Support

Formal support serves four functions: 1) it provides respite for the caregivers; 2) it performs the skilled and sometimes technical aspects of care; 3) it supplies information and reassurance to the caregivers; and 4) it offers spiritual support and counseling. Professional caregivers may also provide emotional support, but this depends on individual personality and cannot be counted on.

To Provide Respite

Respite means a break for the main caregiver from the duties of caregiving. In this respect, formal support can act as a substitute for the main caregiver. Respite can be a few hours a day when an aide comes in and attends to the dying person's personal needs; it can be several hours at night; or it can be up to five days a month during which the patient is placed in a hospice bed in a hospital and the caregiver is given a complete break, although the caregiver may visit frequently at the hospital. Federal regulations for **Medicare** and **Medicaid** state that a dying person is eligible for five in-patient days of respite care every thirty days. If required, this can take place on a monthly basis. Most private insurance policies with a hospice benefit also cover five days a month in-patient respite care. In-patient stays beyond the five consecutive days will not be covered.

A hospice will allot a dying person a set amount of home health aide time per week to be used for respite in whatever form the caregiver decides is most useful. This allotment averages twelve hours a week but may go up to twenty in some hospices. **Continuous care** is the most extensive in home respite care. It is around-the-clock coverage provided by Medicare, Medicaid, and most private insurance companies in cases where pain or symptoms are out of control or when the caregiver is incapacitated. This intense level of coverage rarely lasts longer than seventy-two hours, but it could, in rare cases, extend to four days.

Respite is one of the most important functions that formal support performs, for it can help prevent the primary caregiver from becoming overwhelmed. Because caregivers often delay using formal support until the dying are extremely debilitated and they themselves are on the point of exhaustion, caregivers run the risk of becoming so burdened and so run-down in their own health that they impair their ability to continue caregiving, thereby forcing the dying person back into the hospital or into a nursing home. Pat Knott used formal support in this way:

> We finally got to the point where we were falling apart and we said, "Look, we don't know how much longer this is going to go on. Somehow we have got to protect our own health." We found our insurance would cover some but not all of the expense of having someone come in. So for three weeks before she died, we had someone, someone who came and stayed at night.

Despite Bonnie Steiner's plan to care for David, as a nurse she knew that many unexpected things could occur, and she prepared herself for this:

> I wanted the nurse there just as a support for me. I didn't have any idea of how it was going to get . . . I think I just sort of needed a backup person.

To Provide Skilled Care

Included in skilled care are the services that the registered nurse (RN) performs, such as the initiation of an intravenous line, administration of shots, and performance of nursing assessment. Other professionals who come to the home are social workers and physical therapists. Deciding to have professional services does not mean the caregiver no longer participates in caregiving. The caregiver can choose to be involved in the skilled aspects of care at different levels. Some want to be trained to do all the actual caregiving themselves; they require the services of a nurse to reassure them that they are doing it correctly and to help them solve problems when they arise.

Others want to be present when the skilled care is delivered but do not wish to provide it themselves. Still others want nothing to do with this aspect of care and may choose to remain out of the room when it is delivered. Even when caregivers choose to provide most of the skilled care, reassurance from a nurse is still needed. The following are examples of the ways different informants chose to be involved in the skilled aspects of caregiving. The range extends from Pat Knott, who initially decided to do it all herself, to Lucille De-Mott, who had to have the nurse perform much of Joyce's care while she was at work.

> PAT KNOTT: The home care agency probably could have done some of the things I was doing like changing the dressing, but I think that I felt that no one will do this quite as carefully as I will do it, and once I had been taught how to do it, I was always going to take the time to do it exactly right. If her fist was hyperextended and I was doing range of motion, I would try to get her relaxed and I would keep working at it; whereas someone else would probably have come for thirty minutes and would have done whatever had to be done in that thirty minutes and would have left. So I guess there were things I could have asked people to do, but I was there and I didn't see a reason.

> LUCILLE DEMOTT: I wanted to be involved in all aspects of Jim's care so the VNA [Visiting Nurse Association] nurses even taught me to give him the injections. Other people don't want to be dealing with that at all. The VNA nurses are trained to read the type you are. When they first came in, I was just there and a part of it and that was O.K. Whereas when you are in the hospital, the staff are more apt to try to exclude you from procedures; the given is you don't need to be here. The VNA are well skilled and will include or train the family in procedures if that is desired.

To Supply Information and Reassurance

Although caregivers are comfortable with different degrees of participation in the caregiving process, most require and are extremely grateful for the information and reassurance that professional support can give. Professional support performs two important functions in this respect: 1) it provides caregivers with information concerning the change they can expect to see and the events they can expect to occur as the person dies—something that most informants were unfamiliar with and therefore frightened by; and 2) it reassures caregivers that they are providing the best care possible for their family member. When this is not the case, the professionals intervene to improve the care.

In contemporary U.S. society, many people have little experience with death, and so caregivers are often apprehensive of what will actually occur in death. Its portrayal in movies and television is often gruesome. Accurate information deciphering the signs of approaching death can eliminate or reduce needless anxiety and concern that more could be done to make the patient comfortable (chapter 6 provides this information). Although the physician may describe the death process as something like "slipping into a coma," this description has little to do with what the actual caregiving and problems are likely to be.

Hospitals may make some attempt at letting the caregiver know, when the patient returns home, what can be expected in caregiving and the death process. If the hospital does not do so, the caregiver should ask hospital personnel to describe what to expect. This is one of the most valuable roles hospice performs. Laura Sweet did not have access to hospice or hospital information and reassurance, which caused her and Anthony Lane's parents to suffer needlessly while he was dying.

LAURA SWEET: That night I would have wanted anyone there to explain what was going on. We found out after that his bowel ruptured, so it wasn't necessary for me to be digging him out because I thought I would make him feel better getting this blockage out. He probably wasn't feeling anything at that point. I needed someone to tell us about the pain medicine because his mother was arguing with me and I had to go with my judgment at that point. Right after I gave it to him was when he started breathing funny and I thought I had killed him. We needed medical expertise, someone to just—We were rinsing out dishes, and I was sort of giving orders and trying to make order out of chaos and saying to Tony's father, "Get some more hot water" and trying to make it at least so we weren't all running like chickens with our heads cut off, because that is how we felt. We felt chaotic. Somebody there who could do that other than me so I could just sit there and hold Tony's hand.

I had a feeling that he was dying and I said, "In case I don't see you, goodbye and I love you"—and [I needed] someone to say to me, "For sure, he is really dying," and then I could say everything I wanted to say instead of being tentative about it; so I could really say, "You are dying, and goodbye" and maybe shake his parents up and say, "He is dying. Now is the time to say you love him and goodbye"—Somebody to clean up and I would have much rather concentrated on the feelings of the situation. I guess, for that night, that would have been very helpful.

To Offer Spiritual Support

Spiritual support is available from the clergy and staff associated with a hospice and from the religious institution of which the dying person or caregiver is a member. It is the key element in helping many people cope with the dying process and death. It makes sense out of the often painful and wrenching process and gives caregivers strength to carry on with their caregiving.

Spiritual support takes many forms. Some of the mothers in Pat Knott's church organized a system for providing meals, transportation, and respite for Pat. The clergy visited regularly and prayed with Pat and Don. Members of the congregation prayed frequently with John Wright during his illness, and some gathered for a special silent prayer service with him the day he died. Much to the puzzlement of the grandchildren, Helen and her children gathered around John's bed singing hymns for several hours after he died, which comforted them in their initial grief. One of the stated purposes of hospice is to help people come to terms with their death. Thus it provides professional counseling for the dying person and for the caregiver.

The religious institution of which the dying person and/or caregiver is a member will include the family in its prayers and devotions and will offer spiritual counseling. Depending on the particular organization and the dying person or the caregiver's relationship to it, the support may also include material assistance such as meals, sitting with the patient, and even financial support. Caregivers in need should inquire of their church, temple, or religious organization about possible material support.

The clergy are an invaluable source of information in the planning of the funeral or memorial service. When it is appropriate, they can work with the dying person to tailor these ceremonies to meet individual needs and beliefs.

When the dying person is not a formal member of a congregation, he or she can still call on the clergy for support. Most clergy are willing to respond to the needs of the dying even when no formal relationship exists, which was the case with Elizabeth Krolick.

ANNA KROLICK: Elizabeth hadn't been a member of a church for years, but when she was dying she asked to have the Bible read to her. We did that and prayed with her and thought it would help her to take communion, so we asked the minister from St. Michael's to come. He came several times after that and was really wonderful and patient. We were worried because she hadn't known him and was very hostile to people she didn't know then, but he seemed to know exactly how to handle that problem, and they usually, but not always, got on well.

Deciding to Use Formal Support

Several informants decided on a home death because they wanted to exercise control over the final part of the dying person's life. They did not want this time to be subject to the constraints, routines, and invasions of privacy imposed by the institutional requirements of the hospital. They wanted the person to live as normal a life as possible while dying. Engaging professional services raised some of the same issues of control that these caregivers had encountered in the hospital.

Closely linked to the issue of control and intrusion is that of acceptance of death. Needing help in the home to manage the normal activities of everyday life is an indication that the dying person is weakening. People struggle against the acknowledgment and may deny the need for help long after it is evident. The acceptance of formal services, thus, may symbolize the inevitable approach of death. By talking about patient safety and quality of life, social workers who are aware of the symbolism try to cushion its significance when the topic of hospice is introduced. The significance for most dying people and their caregivers is, however, unavoidable. Many people's reluctance to accept the inevitability of death, which the use of hospice symbolically represents, leads them to forgo services as long as possible.

FLORENCE MARTIN: To get hospice care you have to have a doctor who will say you are terminally ill and will die in six months, and at that point, neither one of us were considering that he would be gone in six months. Hospice will not take you without that certification. He definitely was not ready to see himself as being gone in six months. He finally agreed to it, the month he died.

Fortunately, hospice regulations have changed. A physician now needs to certify only that death is likely in six months if the disease follows its normal course. This flexibility softens the six-month death sentence implied in the former regulations. The family physician is supposed to certify that the patient is eligible for hospice. In cases where the family physician is reluctant to do this, the hospice physician, as a consultant, can make the determination that the patient is terminally ill and eligible for hospice care.

Some families felt that having professional support in the home simply reinforced their agonizing awareness that the person they loved was dying.

Pat Knott felt this acutely:

For some reason I didn't welcome the home care agency. Maybe it was because I didn't feel real close to those people who came from the agency. I had so many people coming at me and I knew I just didn't feel I wanted another stranger. I didn't want to have to explain the story. I remember one time when one woman was there and was asking me what she was like and I felt, "I don't want to tell anybody—I just don't have the energy for this." It was easier to be around the people who knew what she was like and I didn't have to relive that. Because whenever you had to tell somebody what she was like you could see the difference between what she had been like and what she was now. It made me think about it more.

Others accepted the services, believing they had come to terms with the implications of stopping active treatment and accepting the palliative care offered by hospice, but in fact found their understanding changed once the hospice people were actually in the home.

The desire to exercise control over what is left of the dying person's life, and in so doing maintain quality and a kind of normalcy, ironically can contribute to a denial of death. Caregivers are so focused on all the considerable problems involved in maintaining the quality of life and normalcy, which become increasingly difficult as death approaches, that they may lose sight of the fact that death is the outcome for the dying person. Caregiving becomes so overwhelming that it is hard to believe there will be an end to it. In such a delicate situation professional caregivers, if they are strangers, can serve as a painful reminder of what is happening. In some cases, this is welcomed by caregivers and patients because it helps keep them focused on the seriousness of the task and the precious nature of the time left. But others resent the intrusive reminder.

Having formal support inevitably means having strangers in your home. It is difficult to admit strangers both because it is a further acknowledgment of the inevitability of death and because, at such an intensely personal time, strangers are not welcome. Among the cases I studied, sometimes both the dying person and the caregivers had trouble with this. For some of the men who were dying, the outsider represented a threat to their sense of self and to the intimacy of their marital relationship. Initially these men did not want anyone to care for them except their wives.

> LUCILLE DeMOTT: Jim didn't want anyone else to bathe him. He wanted me to bathe him. So when I finally did hire someone, I hired a man, figuring it would be O.K.

As the dying person's condition grew worse, most reservations about outside help usually retreated. Some caregivers continued to have reservations until the death. Florence Martin especially did not want strangers around when her husband died, although she had welcomed their help earlier:

> He definitely felt there was no reason for me to go outside the house. He felt I could hire someone to do the grocery shopping, banking, and so forth. I was never to walk out the door. This made a few problems.
>
> Hospice offered me, when we knew he was dying, to have somebody come out and stay, which I did not want. Because I just really didn't want a stranger here. This was a volunteer type. I just did not want that. I guess . . . I don't know . . . I am funny about things and I guess having a stranger—the idea bothered me.

This is clearly a decision that each family will have to make. Most eventually need outside help. Knowing this, caregivers may wish to consider introducing services before they are absolutely necessary to prevent their own burnout and to ensure the best quality of care for the patient. As we will see in a later section, the family and outside service providers can negotiate issues concerning privacy, and satisfactory solutions can be reached. If outsiders are involved in the care for a sufficiently long time, they cease to be outsiders. In the case of Florence Martin, she did not want the new helpers, people she barely knew, to be present at her husband's death; however, the longtime aide was welcomed. Similarly, Stan Clark desired the presence of the physician and longtime nurse who had cared for his wife, but he found intrusive the new nurse, whom he considered an outsider. Through their participation at such an intimate, intense time in a family's life, professional support people become more than paid caregivers: they often become valued friends, informal family members.

For many caregivers, the decision is clear cut. The dying person is discharged from the hospital in significantly worse condition than when he or she was admitted, and the need for services is obvious and imperative. The ambivalence tends to diminish when the patient is so debilitated as to require almost total care, especially if this is accompanied by some impairment in the ability to communicate.

To summarize, in situations where there is early acknowledgment of the terminal prognosis, services can be introduced into the home as needed. The number of services and their intensity will increase as the patient nears death. The decision to engage professional services is part of the ongoing process of caregiving. It evolves as the patient is dying. Service needs change in response to the dying person's needs, the caregiver's needs, and the changes in informal support. Although it may be difficult to have strangers in the house, their presence from time to time may be essential to make a home death possible.

Assessing the Need for Services

Although the **care plan** will be revised frequently, sometimes continuously as both the caregiver's and the dying person's needs change, it is important to develop some basic understanding of the caregiver's abilities and constraints in caregiving, because it is the main caregiver who will assume the primary responsibility and the major work load by having the patient at home. This assessment is needed to determine where formal support is required and where the caregiver and informal support system can realistically assume responsibility. Formal support, of course, almost always requires payment, and the amount of care needed may not be covered by insurance. In such cases, families can either pay the additional cost themselves or turn to the system of informal support. For specific diseases, additional aid is available from such organizations as the Muscular Dystrophy Society. In other cases, additional volunteer aid may be available from church organizations, or the family may be able to obtain aides from seniors groups at a reasonable hourly rate. The conditions for the availability of this additional support are usually set locally.

The amount and types of services needed depend principally on the physical stamina and psychological well-being of the caregiver, for these will determine the extent to which he or she can cope with competing responsibilities and the functioning of the household.

Many caregivers will be faced with competing responsibilities: children, work, or both. Some people will also be responsible for the care of another sick or dependent person. To the reassuring surprise of many informants, their employers proved flexible in working out arrangements to help them care for the dying person, albeit with some difficulty (these arrangements will be examined in chapter 5). In the care of young children, friends, neighbors, and day care people were similarly flexible and helpful in devising support. The responsibilities of family and work are serious constraints, however, and the response to a request for support may not prove as sympathetic as that encountered by some of the people here. Caregivers need to consider seriously how to manage competing responsibilities so that they are not debilitated by constant additional worry and demands and so that, after the death has occurred, their future lives and well-being, and that of their families, are not jeopardized.

Even—or perhaps especially—when someone is dying and one of the ultimate dramas of life is being played out in the caregiver's home, the work of running a household must go on. When this system falls apart, much more than household order suffers. Although it is clearly more difficult to care for the dying person when there are no clean dishes to use, or the floor is so strewn with debris that passage is difficult, or there is no clean laundry, the real damage is more psychological. People derive security from the order of everyday life. Its sheer repetitiveness is reassuring. In situations such as this, normal everyday life stands in necessary contrast to the destruction being wrought to the fabric of that life. When the simple everyday routines and rituals fail to function, the stress of caregiving increases to intolerable levels.

Caregivers need to consider the basic household tasks and to determine whether someone else can either assume them altogether or offer substantial assistance:

Who does or can do the grocery shopping?
Who does or can do the laundry?
Who gets or can get the children to and from school (if applicable)?
Who cooks or can cook the meals?
Who cleans or can clean the house?
Who cares or can care for yard and house (if applicable)?

Caring for a dying person requires a tremendous amount of physical strength and endurance—as Helena Wolf said, "a Herculean amount of strength." With only one exception, all caregivers were in a state of total exhaustion by the time the patient died. Lucille DeMott was suffering from serious health problems incurred while caring for her husband. The caregiver's ability to care plays some role in the amount of the care prescribed by the dying person's physician; it must be assessed at the outset and reevaluated if the caregiver's physical or mental well-being deteriorates. Caregivers who are themselves ill or debilitated need to consider carefully whether and, if so, how they can assume this responsibility.

Perhaps one of the most crucial questions to ask in assessing the caregiver's stamina is how well the caregiver tolerates lack of sleep or frequently interrupted sleep. Although not all dying people suffer from sleep disturbances, most do at some time, and some do regularly. Chronic sleep deprivation can have serious consequences for the caregiver's physical and emotional well-being and can in itself be sufficient reason for additional professional support. (See appendix A for suggestions regarding this problem.)

Caring for a dying person is simply and clearly an extremely stressful undertaking. No one can be expected to handle this easily. If the prospective caregiver suffers from serious additional psychological problems or limitations, it may be inappropriate for that person even to attempt to take on the responsibility. At the minimum, significant support will be needed.

These factors help predict who will be able to provide care for a dying person, but they are by no means definitive. There are numerous cases in which, through sheer willpower, caregivers surmount extreme problems to care successfully for someone.

Types of Agencies

Although most people associate hospice care with terminal illness, it is not appropriate for all dying people, nor are all dying people able to receive it. Choosing between a home care agency and a hospice will depend on a number of considerations, including the severity of the condition, insurance benefits, the services provided by the different agencies, and the dying person's and caregiver's preference regarding the extent of services desired.

The organization of services offered by a local home care or hospice agency will depend on the training, expertise, and resources of its professionals, its particular organizational structure, the local community's health care system, and state and local regulations. The comparison drawn here is meant to be illustrative, not definitive.

Hospice

Hospice is a philosophy about caring for people who are terminally ill, and it has recently become a specific insurance benefit in Medicare. Many people think of hospice as a lovely place out in the country. This image derives from Britain, where the hospice movement originated and where hospices tend to be in-patient facilities. This is not typically the case in the United States. Although there are in-patient hospice beds at many hospitals and nursing homes and free-standing hospices are being built, Medicare and many other policies with a hospice benefit limit in-patient stays to five days a month. Some policies cover five days or less a month. People do reside longer, but the hospice or hospital will then lose money, which can create tense and difficult situations as the institution begins to urge the patient to leave (or to die—although no one says this outright). A hospice benefit is included in most state Medicaid programs. Exactly which services are covered varies from state to state. Most managed care plans also include this benefit, and, again, the plans vary in terms of which services are covered.

The hospice philosophy advocates the provision of care for the pain and symptoms associated with dying. This is called palliative care. Hospice will not take any action to prolong life. The hospice physician will treat easily managed conditions or symptoms. Programs may differ on what will be treated, and this should be discussed before engaging their services. Hospice recognizes the need for care that supports the informal, family care system and offers a wider range of services than traditional home care. Some hospices are organized as agencies similar to home care agencies and may in fact be part of such an agency. Others operate as consultant teams and subcontract the actual care to home care agencies, but in addition they provide special hospice supervision and backup and other services not customarily found in a home care agency.

For hospice care, the physician must certify that the person is likely to die within six months if the disease takes its normal course. A potential drawback in accepting hospice care concerns the involvement of the person's physician. Once a patient is in the hospice program, the reimbursement for the physician is limited to home visits made. If the doctor is reluctant to make such visits, the patient will either be seen by a physician associated with the hospice agency or will have to pay **out-of-pocket** for the visits of the personal physician. This prospect may be especially upsetting for people who, in the process of fighting their disease, have developed a close relationship with their physician. If a person selects hospice, the doctor may continue to remain involved in care by signing prescriptions and maintaining phone contact even though he or she does not visit the home. In this way the patient need not feel abandoned. It is important to note that the patient's physician can be reimbursed for his or her services as long as the treatment consists of symptom or pain management and not aggressive therapy. For example, a patient suffering from AIDS may continue to use his or her AIDS specialist to manage conditions associated with AIDS. The hospice reimbursement specialist will help the physician "capture" the reimbursement and the family should encourage the physician to seek this assistance. The physician can either bill the patient's insurance directly or bill hospice, which will in turn help the physician "capture" the reimbursement.

According to the National Hospice Association (Kilburn 1988), hospice differs from home care in the following ways:*

1. *Hospice provides central case management and continuity of care between home and in-patient settings.* Hence someone in the hospice will oversee the different aspects of the dying person's care, relieving the caregiver of the burden of management. It also attempts to maintain **continuity of care** between the in-patient (hospital or nursing

---

*These criteria apply to Medicare-certified hospices. If a hospice is not certified by Medicare, it does not have to offer this range of benefits.

home) and home settings. This particular function is one of the most important aspects of hospice care, for it means that the hospice will take responsibility for making sure a staff person is in the home when expected by the caregiver. In other words, if, for instance, an aide can't show up, the hospice will make sure the caregiver is relieved by someone else. In caring for the terminally ill, dependability of relief for caregivers is essential.

2. *A hospice utilizes a team model of care,* which means that a physician, social worker, nurse, often a chaplain, and others such as a dietician, physical therapist, and other auxiliary health care professionals collaborate in care. This facilitates a smooth approach and good communication among the different people caring for the dying person.

3. *Hospice has additional services not traditionally offered,* such as volunteers to help support the family and care for the patient, bereavement counseling after the person has died, support groups for families, spiritual care, and more involvement with the patient's hospice physician.

4. *Hospice focuses on the caregiver and caregiving family as well as on the dying person.*

5. *Hospice services are available on a twenty-four-hour basis, seven days a week.* This intense level of service is available only in times of crisis, and its necessity must be certified by a physician for hospice to be reimbursed. The kinds of services available at this level include nursing and physician contact and the possibility of visits to the home, prescription drugs, and medical supplies and equipment. In addition, people who staff the hospice during off-hours are familiar with the individuals cases and can communicate and report to the appropriate team members.

6. *Hospice has the authority to place the dying person in an in-patient setting* to improve symptom control, to provide the caregivers with a respite, or as a permanent move if care burdens overwhelm the caregivers.

7. *Hospice team members are especially trained in pain control methods and in working with the terminally ill and their families.*

8. *Hospice includes in the care plan the combined physical, social, emotional, and spiritual needs of the family as well as the dying person.*

9. *Hospice offers bereavement counseling on an as-needed basis for thirteen months after the death has taken place.*

With its explicit philosophy of acknowledging and assisting in death, hospice makes dying very much an active part of its care. For example, Helen Wright said the hospice workers were good "at reminding John that he was dying, even though he knew it, to remind him to say something if he wanted to say it. 'Do you have anything to say to Helen? You want to be able to say what you want to say.' 'Well,' he says, 'we've been in pretty good touch for the last twenty years. I don't think I have any more to say.'" Sometimes, in the process of helping dying people and their families come to terms with death, hospice workers can intrude into areas that the dying person or family wish to remain private. When this happens the people concerned need to put limits on the hospice worker's involvement, as did John Wright.

Hospice philosophy is demonstrated in a different style of care, in which attention is focused on making the dying person comfortable, not on helping him or her regain health. Well-trained hospice workers should be sensitive to the extreme strain the caregiver is under and be especially flexible in meeting needs as they arise.

LUCILLE DeMOTT: When you have a nurse or aide who is not hospice trained, then he or she is trained to complete the physician's orders. So in Jim's case one order states he is to take particular pills at specific times. When he got to the point where he couldn't swallow pills, some private duty nurse then gave them to him while I was asleep. It was stupid; she tried to crumble them, which made it worse because he couldn't swallow all those little lumps. We ended up calling someone with suction equipment in the middle of the night to handle the problem. I found that rigid adherence to orders among RNs all the time, whereas people who were hospice trained accepted that this person was going to die and that the important issue was good quality of life. A pill at four o'clock was not important at this point in his life; whereas hospice-trained nurses were sensitive and flexible, other RNs followed doctors' orders. Boy, they follow doctors' orders—not always very sensibly.*

An additional factor that differentiates a hospice from a home care agency is the team focus. Although many dying people and their

---

*Lucille DeMott is describing three kinds of professional caregivers: aides, who have minimal training but can be taught by the caregiver to perform certain tasks; registered nurses (RNs) and licensed practical nurses (LPNs), who are sent by an agency but have no hospice training; and hospice-trained RNs and LPNs, who are experienced in caring for the dying.

families appreciate this comprehensive approach to care, some do not want to relate to all the different team members. They consider the extra people an intrusion.

The spiritual approach of hospice differentiates it from a home care agency. Research shows that the people who work for hospice are highly motivated and committed to their job. Hospice employees and volunteers often are involved in the organization because of their own religious beliefs. This integrated approach can be very reassuring to and supportive of the dying person and caregiver. The terminally ill and their families who do not share a spiritual approach to life and death, however, may not welcome it at such a difficult time in their lives.

> LUCINDA KLEIN: Every single nurse, including the one we got along with, was always carrying a Bible. They would sit there and read it. Joyce said, "You make me feel like I am dead already and you are praying over me. I don't want this in my house; leave me alone." That was a weird thing, that was really kind of icky.

If spiritual counseling is *not* desired by the patient, the caregiver can request that it not be given.

The hospice agency receives a flat fee of $107.68 a day from Medicare or $107.82 from Medicaid (according to 1997 guidelines). This fee must cover all the services and drugs the dying person requires. A hospice may be reluctant to accept patients who require heavy or extensive, around-the-clock care because it will be difficult for them to cover their expenses. This is more of a problem for the smaller, privately run hospices than for the larger ones with greater access to funds. The hospice prefers to accept patients several months before they are expected to die, so that it can build up surplus funds when the dying person requires relatively little care. This surplus can later be used when the care needs become more intensive. Volunteers are used to fill gaps in service created by heavy-demand patients. It is important to ask an agency about the availability of volunteers.

Hospices should never turn down a patient because of inability to pay. The caregiver should request that the hospice's indigent care fund be used to cover the costs and should talk with the hospice social worker to evaluate whether the patient is eligible for Medicaid. It is not ethical for a hospice to turn down a patient.

Home Care

Often home care agencies have a hospice component. When they do not, it is important to examine carefully the range of services which they offer. Many local agencies offer a fuller range of services—for example, pastoral care and social work—than is found in the large national home care chains. These local agencies may combine hospice and home care services, a combination that allows them to offer basically the same range of services to all clients and simply to assign the dying person to either the hospice or home care benefit depending on which is to the financial advantage of the agency and the individual. Local agencies are able to do this because they can attract volunteers and because they may have patient care funds, donated in memory of their patients, which help offset deficits. These agencies, however, may lack the level of expertise necessary to oversee highly technical home care, for which one may have to turn to the local branch of a national agency.

The Medicare home care benefit, which tends to be more restrictive than private insurance, will pay for a higher, more intense level of services for a longer period than hospice. These must be skilled services (e.g., injections, wound dressing, assessments, initiation and maintenance of a catheter, and IV initiation and maintenance), however, performed by a nurse. If the condition is not judged serious enough to require skilled care, the agency's bill for payment may not be certified, so agencies must be careful when they provide this level of care and are reluctant to do so except when it is clearly needed. In addition, Medicare requires that the patient pay 20 percent of the cost of medications.*

Health Maintenance Organization

If the dying person is a member of a **health maintenance organization (HMO)**, the caregiver's choice will be limited. Many HMOs—by no means all—have a hospice benefit. As a member, however, the dying person will have to receive care from the home care or hospice agency with which the HMO has a contract. It may or may not be a good agency, but unless the patient or caregiver is willing to pay for the care privately, this is the only choice available. When a hospice

---

* Because of the frequent changes in reimbursement policy and the attempts to expand the coverage for home care, a caregiver needs to inquire about current reimbursement guidelines when calling a home agency or hospice.

benefit is not available, the caregiver should appeal to the **case manager** to get permission to go out of the system. If hospice care is cost effective, which it usually is, the case manager will have the HMO cover the services. If this is allowed, it is likely that the choice will be limited to certified hospices, thus excluding the local home care agencies that sometimes function as hospices.

The HMO restriction is primarily a problem for those who do not qualify for Medicare (primarily people under sixty-five) and for the small but growing number of Medicare recipients who belong to a Medicare HMO.

A hospice offers a wide range of services for the terminally ill and their families. To be accepted for hospice, the dying person does not have to pay for medications but usually cannot immediately have heavy care needs. The local home care agency may offer the same wide range of services as the hospice but be available to people requiring heavy care; here the patient is responsible for 20 percent of the costs of the medication. An affiliate of a national home care corporation will probably not offer a wide range of support services but will have the expertise to maintain a person who requires the use of sophisticated medical technology in order to remain at home. In fact, many large home care chains are hesitant to accept dying patients because of the heavy care demands they represent and the agencies' inability to guarantee the patient's safety without providing additional staff and resources, for which they may not receive compensation. An exception to this preference occurs when a long-time agency patient is dying and requests to remain with the agency and the same staff: in many such cases, considerable effort is made to meet the needs of the patient.

Professionals Who Work in the Home

Although the regulations governing hospice are less stringent than those for home care, reimbursement regulations will determine the kind and extent of care available to the dying person and family. The regulations tend to be rather rigid. It is important to understand how they work, in order to avoid potential conflicts with the agency and to plan for informal care to supplement that which is reimbursable. This section, in addition to identifying the activities for which the professional can be reimbursed, describes the role each type played in the care of the people in this study.

Physicians

Having a good relationship with a dying person's physician is extremely important for the effective delivery of care and for the patient's well-being. A physician who is involved in the care can monitor the effectiveness of the various medications and procedures and help control and alleviate the symptoms of the terminal disease, as well as attend to the health of the caregiver. The doctor's role, however, is not clearly defined and varies considerably according to the individual's temperament and commitment. For reimbursement purposes, a physician must oversee the care of each home care and hospice patient. This means that he or she must participate in a minimum of one monthly interdisciplinary team meeting to review individual patient care plans. Many agencies require more than one monthly meeting. Caregivers who wish to bring up a care problem should find out when these meetings are held and ask that the problem be discussed at the team meeting.

In many cases, the dying person's physician withdraws from active involvement in the person's care, at least in part because few are trained in such care. There are few role models and little specific information. Dying people and those who care for them cannot know what to anticipate from their physician until the patient is no longer receiving treatment and is seen to be dying. Half the people in this book had very good experiences with their physicians. The others were ambivalent or had poor experiences.

HELENA WOLF: The physician would come by, I guess once or twice, and we would have these discussions about "well, what do you think, how long do you think he has, what do you expect to see?" and he was always very vague. I don't know if he was very vague because he didn't know or because he didn't want to alarm us, but to some extent I felt relatively abandoned at least by the professional community: I didn't feel that I got a whole lot of support from them.

Symptom management is where I feel the physician really let us down. I eventually had to call him and say, "Lookit, Herbert seems to be awfully agitated and isn't there something we could do?" He had given me some Valium. I said, "Could we give some to Herbert?" He said, "Oh sure, that would be a good idea," and that kind of stuff and never saying, "Let's take a look at this," and "Here are some ways you could handle this."

Other informants were more fortunate in their relations with physicians, who were able to accept that their patient was dying and to continue to provide support to both patient and family.

STAN CLARK: The physician was concerned with where to put the couch, so people could sit comfortably there and still be in the room with Alice, and how to handle the phone for her. He was involved in all aspects of Alice's care, her quality of life, her comfort, and always there when I needed him.

LUCILLE DEMOTT: I am convinced that if you want home doctor visits you can get them. You may have to change doctors, but, if that is an important item on your list of how you want to manage your home care, they do exist and can be very, very helpful. Our particular physician was helpful because he spent a lot of time with me and always inquired how I was doing during his home visits.

ANNA KROLICK: My mother was very agitated. We had tremendous trouble finding something to give her to calm her down but not knock her out. Her doctor was great. He was always available by phone. Either he or one of his fellows would call us right back. He told us to call him at home any time we needed him. It was very reassuring to know he was there and it was extremely important to her to know he hadn't abandoned her.

Efforts are being made to train physicians to care better for dying patients. These are just beginning, however, and there are many doctors who have great difficulty treating the dying. If involvement with a physician is important, caregivers need to make an effort to seek one out who is capable of treating the dying. The physicians who work with hospices, by choice, participate in this care and tend to be very sympathetic to the needs of patient and family.

Caregivers who wish to find a compatible physician can do so by calling different agencies, hospitals, and other physicians and asking for a referral to someone who cares for terminally ill, homebound patients. A certified hospice already has an affiliation with such a physician. Caregivers will need to know the answers to the following kinds of questions in advance, before a crisis arises:

What is the physician's philosophy of pain control (if appropriate)?
Is someone always on call for the doctor?
Does she or he make house calls?
Will the physician attend to the caregiver (if appropriate)?
Will the doctor work with the home care or hospice agency the
     caregiver has selected?

Nurses

Visits from nurses are for skilled nursing assessment and for treatments such as wound care, change of dressings, and IV treatment. The visits can also include teaching the caregiver how to care for the patient. If there is an aide providing personal care to the patient, the nurse will supervise the aide. The number of hours a nurse can visit a week is determined by the level of care the dying person requires.

Nurses who are skilled in the care of the dying are particularly valuable for the advice they can provide. Caring for someone who is dying requires making numerous small and large decisions and solving small and large problems. A skilled nurse can provide assistance in this area. Lucille DeMott was particularly impressed by the skill of the nurses she worked with compared to that of the home health aides:

> In my experience, the aides were pretty good in doing specific tasks once you worked with them and made sure you were getting what you wanted. They were not skilled at making suggestions at improving things. We needed skilled care and used both RNs and LPNs. What was astounding to me was [that] an RN would come and make five good suggestions which had not occurred to me before. It was certainly worth paying that person's wage just in terms of improved care because a pro knew something. Once you have the system set up with the lowest-level agency person, I would have an RN come in and critique how it is working and suggest better ways of doing it.

Most people in this book felt that home care and hospice nurses provided excellent care and substantial support for the caregiver and family. One valuable role that nurses can play is in obtaining information and cooperation from the physician. Good communication between the nurse and doctor is an essential aspect of good, quality care and an important reason to ask the physician for a referral to the home care or hospice agency he or she uses.

> JOE STEAD: The home care nurse called the first night we were with the agency, and she talked with me—nicest person in the world. She told me what she could do and what they would like to do and she would try and wanted to know the doctor's name, and I told her, so she checked with the doctor. She talked with the doctor and the doctor thought we understood that Dorothy wouldn't live. Now thinking back, the last time we were there, the doctor said, "Mrs. Stead, we can't give you any more chemo or it will kill you." And from that—she didn't say she was going to die—you know how my hopes are going to be, so I didn't think of it that way. Well, I would take care of her as long as I could.

Nurses are also trained to deal with the psychosocial problems that confront the dying person and the family.

Caregivers tend to use nurses supplied by the home care or hospice agency. The caregiver has a right to interview the nurse in advance, at which time it should be determined whether the nurse would be compatible with the family and the patient. In addition, the caregiver should seek information in the following areas:

Will the nurse provide continuity of care by being the one person to decide how procedures should be done?
Will the nurse supervise the aides, and how closely?
Is the nurse familiar with the dying person's special needs?
Who will be on call for the nurse?

Home Health Aides

An aide is the person who comes into the home to provide personal care for the dying person. Usually the aide's visits are two hours long. During this time the aide can change the bed, clean up the room, prepare a meal, do a little washing. The aide is there primarily to care for the patient's personal needs and secondarily to help the family. The aide *cannot* administer medications.

The home health aide provides the kind of care most families need when caring for a dying person: relieving the caregiver from the unremitting strain of interacting with and caring for someone who is dying. Unfortunately, reimbursement for this service is very limited. If the family feels they need more than the allotted two hours a day of home health aide care, for example, if the main caregiver is sick, they should ask for this additional help. Anna Krolick's family felt they could not have cared for their mother without the help of their aide, Thelma. Because her help was so significant, they all contributed to pay her salary beyond the two hours a day paid for by Medicare. This cost of her care was determined on a sliding scale based on Elizabeth's ability to pay, not that of her children.

> ANNA KROLICK: When the nurse asked us if we wanted an aide, I didn't know what to say, what an aide could do. Now I don't think I could have done it without her. She sat in the room with my mother and turned her and bathed her, but mostly was a calm, comforting presence. My mother loved her. When we were around, even though we did all the real care, my mother was tense; she could feel our anxiety and grief and it wasn't restful for her. That is what she told Thelma. With Thelma she could let go and cry or pray or whatever. We rarely left the house, but just being able to leave the room was an immense relief.

Other Professionals

There are many different kinds of services that can come to the home. Some are reimbursable. Physical therapy, occupational therapy, recreational therapy, and the technicians and equipment needed (e.g., a mechanical ventilator) for providing technological care at home are reimbursable if ordered by a physician. A caregiver can privately hire an attendant to sit with the patient. The caregiver can also request that the hospital send out a physical therapist to teach the caregiver body mechanics to prevent injuries while pulling and lifting the patient. This should be covered by insurance. A social worker or psychiatrist can come if the physician makes a referral and if one can be located who will make home visits. In some cases, pharmacists and laboratory technicians who draw blood will make home visits. These need to be individually arranged and are not standard practice. When someone is dying, other professionals, among them bankers and lawyers, may make home visits if asked.

Gaining Access to the Formal System

Access through Discharge from the Hospital

Obtaining professional support can be a complex process. If the dying person is leaving the hospital, the discharge planner—someone, often a nurse, who is responsible for arranging the services the patient will receive outside the hospital—and the attending physician will determine the amount of home care required. This determination is crucial, for it decides the amount of reimbursed costs the person is entitled to. With the help of the discharge planner, the caregiver must also select an agency, evaluate how much the dying person's insurance can pay and how much he or she can pay out-of-pocket, and select the type and mixture of services most suited to the caregiver and the patient's needs.

In Lucinda Klein's case the discharge planner greatly facilitated the move home:

> The social worker at the hospital did everything. She contacted the Human Resources Administration, a portion of it called the Crisis Intervention Unit, which handles home care for AIDS patients who have Medicaid, and between the two of them, she just ordered all the equipment and supplies which we needed and ones we didn't need. When we made suggestions of additional things, she added those things, and they delivered it. Joyce came home on a Monday and they delivered it on the Friday before and set it up so there was really nothing I needed to do in terms of that at all. It's all pretty straightforward.

With the changes in reimbursement that give hospitals a financial incentive to discharge patients as soon as possible, discharge planning has become an integrated part of almost every hospital stay. Discharge planning is a process that begins as soon as the patient is admitted. Hospitals are under pressure from insurance companies and Medicare to move patients out as soon as possible. If a patient remains in the hospital beyond a certain point that has been established for each diagnosis, the hospital loses money. Thus the hospital has a strong incentive to help families to begin planning for home care from the very beginning. If the reason for the hospitalization is very traumatic, however, such that it is difficult for the caregiver to think beyond the immediate present, the discharge planner will have to wait until the patient is stabilized and the caregiver can begin thinking about discharge. It can be beneficial for all concerned if the caregiver is involved in this process early.

Importantly, if the discharge planner is aware that the caregiver is trying to work out a care plan but is experiencing difficulty, he or she can mediate between the family, which needs more time, and the hospital administration, which seeks an early discharge (see chapter 1). The effectiveness of this service depends on how well the hospital is organized and on the skills of the individual planner; furthermore, some departments within hospitals have better discharge planning than others.

It sometimes happens that the family and hospital disagree about the patient's fitness for discharge. In some cases, as with the Krolicks in chapter 1, the family might simply require more time to make the arrangements for home care. If the physician knows the family is actively engaged in making these arrangements, he or she may be willing to allow the patient to remain in the hospital longer. But when the family feels the dying person is simply too sick to go home and the hospital staff believe they no longer can do anything to improve the patient's condition, problems develop. Caregivers who want to have the person die at home will have to accept that the patient may not get any better or even stabilize, and that, if they want home death, they must take the patient home despite the seriousness of the condition. If this seems an impossible undertaking, then the caregiver, the physician, and the discharge planner need to consider nursing home placement. It is important for caregivers to understand, however, that this is something that can be negotiated. The hospital cannot discharge the patient until a safe discharge plan has been developed.

The discharge planner will work with the home care agency or hospice to begin establishing a system of care before the dying person leaves the hospital. During the hospital stay, both the caregiver and the patient will assist in assessing their needs and designing the plan. The effectiveness and appropriateness of this system, however, depends on the abilities of the discharge planner and agency, the accuracy of the caregiver's own assessment of the situation, and the stability of the dying person's condition. If this planning is not done in the hospital, the agency nurse will establish a care plan soon after the patient is discharged.

ANNA KROLICK: When I was in the hospital, I had a very minimal idea of how much support I would need. They kept telling me it would be difficult, but no one ever explained how difficult. I thought maybe two to three days a week or several hours a morning. The afternoon we brought her home, the agency nurse was there waiting for us. She helped us map out a plan for how much care we would need. She just assumed we would need full-time, five-days-a-week care. At first I was going to say no, but she said it was better for their scheduling if they started high and then cut back if I didn't need it. By the next day I was very grateful for the help. It could have been seven days a week.

If the dying person remains at home for some time before death, or if no major hospitalization is involved during the last phase of life, the care needs will increase as death approaches and the care plan will have to be changed. If an agency is helping to care for the patient, it should participate in changing these plans. The caregiver will also be expected to participate in this planning process by assessing his or her own needs and changes in the family's ability to care. The agency's role here is essential, for the stressed caregiver often does not even know what to ask for.

The agency, either hospice or home care, will develop a plan for organizing care. At a minimum, this refers to the schedule of visits by the nurses, home health aides, and any other professionals involved in caregiving from that agency. It also includes the times informal caregivers will help. The plan will also detail the schedule of medication and the schedule of other interventions such as turning the person, giving liquids, changing dressings. Care plans can become quite elaborate, especially when they include a number of different informal caregivers.

The point of the planning process is to determine whether the dying person can safely return home. The discharge planner will review the patient's insurance policy to see what kind of coverage is available for home care. The home care benefit, which pays for professional support services, varies greatly from policy to policy. (The financing of home care will be discussed in greater detail later in this chapter.) Once the limits for reimbursed care are known, the discharge planner and, often, the physician will work with the caregiver and the family to decide whether they are able to care for the patient. They may interview the potential caregivers carefully and seek firm commitments of exactly how much care those family members and others besides the main caregiver are willing to provide. Someone from the home care agency or hospice that will care for the patient may visit the home to determine whether the physical setting can accommodate caregiving and whether those living there are capable of participating in the care.

In certain cases, the discharge planner will suggest that the agency nurse come into the hospital to assess the dying person and the caregiver. When there is concern on the part of either the caregiver, the discharge planner, or the physician about the caregiver's ability to care for the patient at home, the discharge planner may ask the caregiver to move into the hospital for twenty-four hours and participate in the care for the dying person. This will either help strengthen the caregiver's confidence or suggest that some other solution is more realistic.

The discharge planner will usually provide a list of possible agencies, and the caregiver must then contact them and decide which to choose. In many cases, the hospitals have formal or informal arrangements with agencies that may be run by former staff members, and there may be subtle or not so subtle attempts to steer the caregiver toward these. Although they may be excellent, it is a good idea to call all the agencies on the list and to compare the cost and range of services. This is also true when the hospital runs its own agency. Some—unfortunately rare—hospitals practice continuity of care and have the nurse who cared for a patient in the hospital follow that same patient at home. Such an arrangement, if available, is a powerful incentive to select the hospital agency. In most cases, however, the hospital agency has no inherent advantages over outside ones. In some instances, hospital-based agencies suffer from poor management because they are so distinctly different from the hospital organization that manages them.

Access without Prior Hospitalization

When seeking a home care agency or hospice without the aid of a discharge planner, there are several approaches to take. The personal physician, if the dying person has one, may be able to recommend an agency with which she or he frequently works. This arrangement has advantages for enhancing the quality of care, for it facilitates quick and efficient communication between the nurses caring for the patient and the doctor. A close working relationship with a physician is extremely important when pain control is at stake, for it facilitates adequate and timely pain relief.

Not all physicians are helpful in this regard. Many have doubts about the quality of care available in the home and are reluctant to refer to or work with a home care agency. If the dying person has no personal physician or if the physician offers little assistance, the caregiver can call the local Visiting Nurse Association or the social work department at a local hospital and ask for a list of local agencies.

Contacting an Agency

Preparations

Before making telephone calls to and visiting prospective agencies, prepare a list of questions and collect information about the patient's care needs and insurance coverage. A notebook for recording the information about the different agencies is an invaluable aid.

The caregiver must have the relevant facts concerning the patient's insurance coverage handy, for the first questions most agencies ask have to do with insurance. Often a caregiver's first contact with an agency occurs during an extremely stressful time, possibly soon after being told there is nothing more the hospital can do and the family member's death is inevitable. To be asked about ability to pay at such a time seems insensitive to many caregivers. Yet the agencies must ask, because they are businesses. Although some will have a sliding scale for people who have difficulty paying, they will first want to explore all possible avenues of reimbursement. The details of insurance are needed regardless of ability to pay. The hospital discharge planner can help to provide this information and in some cases may make these initial contacts for the caregiver.

Questions to Ask

Ask questions about staffing and reimbursement for services. Although these may be asked over the telephone, a visit to each agency to gather this basic information provides considerable additional knowledge about the quality of the agency and the type of staff it employs.

Staffing

General

Will the same nurse or home health aide visit the home every time?
What about emergencies at night and during the weekend?
Will I be guaranteed a substitute if the nurse or aide does not show up?
If I need help when my regular nurse or aide is not available, will the person who comes be familiar with the case?

Nurses

What is the average length of a nursing visit?
Does the nurse have time for the family or just for the patient?
Can we meet and interview the nurse and home health aide in advance?
Can we change nurses if there is a problem?

Aides

Who will organize the schedule of aides in the home?
Will I have to hire the aides myself, or does the agency do this?
Who will oversee the aide's work?
Can I switch aides if there is a problem?
How long are the aide's visits?
Can the agency provide a specific list of duties that the aide is supposed to perform?

Reimbursement

Will the agency provide a list of the charges for all services in advance?
Which services are covered and which are not?
Does the agency have a sliding scale and a patient care fund? (See page 69, "Preparations.")
(If applicable) Will the agency accept Medicaid?
(If in an HMO) Is there a hospice benefit? What services are covered by it? What is the extent of services available?

Miscellaneous

Does the agency have a supply of durable medical equipment to loan patients?
When dealing with a non-hospice home care agency, ask if the agency staff will support end-of-life requests by the dying person—for example, that 911 not be called.

Does the agency offer or have connections to other services, such as
psychiatrists or social workers?
Does the agency offer volunteer services?
Is spiritual support offered?

Supervision

Perhaps the most important questions the caregiver needs to ask are
those concerning supervision and backup coverage. In most of the
cases presented here, the serious problems that arose in dealing with
professional caregivers could be attributed to the inadequate supervision and the inability of the agency to provide adequate backup
coverage. The caregiver is too preoccupied and stressed with responsibilities to assume the chore of supervising the outside help.
Despite the best intentions, problems arise, sometimes serious ones,
and the agency must be ready to supervise its workers and take
responsibility for solving these problems. Likewise, even the most
reliable aides may sometimes be unable to come as planned, and the
agency must provide substitute personnel. Here are some examples
of the kinds of problems a caregiver can encounter when the supervision is not adequate:

> LUCILLE DeMOTT: Many people come into your home, and they are
> coming into an intensely private, emotional time in your life where
> everyone is walking on eggs. We did whatever we could do to try to
> maintain normalcy in the family. We continued our candlelight dinners
> and our birthday parties. Even though we did so many things to at least
> give the image of having a normal life, we were not *having* a normal life.
> Routines, thoughts, and reactions are very skewed; so the people who
> come into your home under those conditions really don't know how to
> get into that fabric. It is a rare person probably who can integrate herself
> into the family. I am sure people could be trained if we worked on it.
>
> One person who came in was very good in some ways; but she
> would come in, in her bathing suit, and unless Jim needed her, she
> would lay out in the yard in a skimpy bikini sunbathing. We were
> paying her a lot of money that we couldn't really afford, and it was one
> of those situations where you ordinarily would nip it in the bud and
> say, "This is inappropriate." But you don't. There must have been five
> adults walking around and no one ever said anything. But how could a
> person be so crass as to do something like that when you are dealing
> with your life fabric being taken from you?

There was no supervision of home care workers in the home. I would never hire them again without insisting that the agency come to the home on surprise visits. There needs to be some kind of supervision. The system is designed so that you are supposed to inform the agency whether you are happy or not, and you are not able to manage that on top of everything else when you think they are there to help you. It is just one too many things to manage.

HELENA WOLF: Hospice theoretically managed the aides. When they came from the agency, there was a supervisor, but I was not impressed by any of them. We had one woman who came during the day, who hospice got for us, who bathed my father, and sat and talked and she was good. My father liked her. She gave me a real break, and I could go off and do some of my own stuff.

The people who were there at night were not so good. I could go and sleep in my own bed; but whenever anything happened in the night, they would come and call me so I was up and down all during the night. I didn't feel that they were very sensitive at all. Herbert was not very happy about them either. He was happy someone was there and he could see that I was at least getting a little sleep, but I think given his druthers he would have rather had me there. He complained that they would fall asleep. He would wake up and they were asleep.

LAURA SWEET: We called hospice, and I told the woman we thought Tony was dying. We had contacted hospice before this—it wasn't just a call out of the blue. "We think he is dying and we don't know what to do." She said, "What's going on?" I said, "His pulse is 140 and has been that way for a few hours; he is very cold and clammy." This is before all that stuff started coming out of him. He had lost his ability to walk, and I said, "Do you know, can you tell if he is going to die?" And she said, "It could be days," and that is not true with all those symptoms. And she said, "What do you want me to do?" I said, "We want some kind of reassurance." She said, "There is really nothing I can do." She said, "You don't really want me to come out there, do you?" I said, "I don't know." She said, "Just give me a call back later and we'll see," or something, and wound up the conversation and said, "Just keep doing what you are doing."

And so I just hung up. We found out later that this particular woman had to catch a flight at five in the morning so she probably didn't want to get involved and probably shouldn't have been on duty. It is a volunteer service, and these people are not as dedicated as paid professionals, maybe. Anyway, that was bad; she could have told us that he was dying and there really was no need to go through all this stuff that we were going through.

Perhaps these problems could have been prevented if the workers involved had been adequately supervised. Workers in people's homes operate with considerable individual discretion. Supervision can, however, help identify potential problems and change the situation to prevent their recurrence or introduce new arrangements to correct them.

Finding the Right People

Even though the agency one has selected may be well recommended and fit the needs of the dying person and family, this does not guarantee that the people who come to the home, the nurse and home health aide in particular, will be compatible with the caregiver and the patient. Most agencies will allow clients to change the staff in the home if there are any personality conflicts. If the agency will not allow this, it may indicate that it is not appropriate for the needs of a dying person. Most of the people described here switched staff or agencies at least once; some changed several times until they established a satisfactory working relationship with the staff in the home. The caregiver and dying person are the clients in this situation. They have a right to demand satisfaction, to have their needs met. If this is not happening, they should consider changing agencies. Vigilance over the quality of care the dying person receives is a valuable contribution that the caregiver can make to that care.

LUCILLE DeMOTT: One of the aspects of caregiving where you should have some certainty is that the person coming into your home will fit into a very stressful situation. The only way you can do it is through interviewing the people agencies recommend ahead of time, then working with those you select to show them what you want.

PAT KNOTT: We called many different agencies and finally settled on a particular agency. They said they would send someone out starting Monday; and we said, "No you don't understand: we will interview someone to decide whether we want that person to come into our home." This was a very foreign idea to them; they didn't want to waste their people's time by coming out. To me it just made sense that, if someone is coming into your house and caring for your sick child, you want to get a feeling for them. So we actually did interview two or three people; and one in that short time got very attached to Lisa.

LAURA SWEET: The home care agency was great, very accommodating. There were a couple of nurses we didn't feel comfortable with; and we asked them not to come back and felt bad. But the bottom line was, "This is Tony's home and we want to be comfortable in this house." But some of the nurses were so wonderful. One would bake goodies and another had defrosted my fridge and cleaned cabinets. It was such a relief to me.

The need to ensure the quality of the aides who care for the dying person is even greater if the caregiver will not be home all the time. Any sick person, but especially one who is dying, is vulnerable. Although agencies make an effort to screen their employees, abuses do happen.

Unfortunately, it is not always possible to obtain a good fit, at least not initially. The agency may simply not have adequate personnel to choose among. Certain times, like nights, are so difficult to staff that the family must accept whoever is available or make do themselves. Sometimes these problems can be overcome by training the staff person; sometimes the caregiver simply must do without adequate assistance.

LUCILLE DeMOTT: The hospital gave me a list of agencies to call, but basically the deciding issue becomes which agency has someone who could come [for] desirable hours. Instead of finding an aide to fit the family and the house, it became, which one or two available people did you want.

ANNA KROLICK: I was so exhausted I had to get some sleep, and my husband was out of town. We tried to get some help at night. What a disaster! The woman was loud and sort of gross. My mother was very agitated then and kept **hallucinating** and this woman insisted on talking to her rationally. She kept upsetting Elizabeth and wouldn't change no matter what I said. I finally sent her home about 2 A.M. and just dealt with it. I was so incredibly disappointed.

There are times when the staff of the agency are so inappropriate or irresponsible that the caregiver has no choice but to change agencies. This experience is traumatic. The family does, however, have the right to change agencies and to find one that better fits its needs, except if the dying person's insurance is with an HMO, in which case reimbursed care will be limited to the HMO-approved agency, and the caregiver will have to protest vigorously to the HMO administration.

Lucille DeMott was forced to change agencies after one disastrous experience:

> When I finally did hire someone, I hired a man, figuring it would be O.K. Everything went very smoothly until Memorial Day weekend. I liked the young man; Jim liked him. The fellow was working more hours than he said he wanted to, so I said, "Memorial Day weekend is coming up. Do you want time off? The agency could find someone else." He said, "No I want to work." So I said O.K. On the first morning of this four-day weekend this guy doesn't show up. I got a call from a friend of his saying he had car trouble. I called the agency and told them. They asked if he would be there or not; I didn't know. They didn't know if they could find someone. Later in the day a friend of the aide's called looking for him. He said the aide was out partying and he had taken his car without asking. I called the agency and informed them of this call, and they told me it was my fault because I was working him too many hours and that he was tired and just needed some time off, and if he hadn't needed time off, this wouldn't have happened. It was not a good scene.
>
> Under those circumstances you change agencies. So we went to a different agency run by a woman whose husband had died. She decided to establish an agency because she was astounded at how poor home care was. Her people were very good.

There are many things a caregiver can do to make sure the quality of care received from professional caregivers is as good as possible. Many home health aides are not very well trained, nor do they have any special ability to care for the dying. In such cases caregivers may need to help train the aide in the specific tasks that need to be done.

> LUCILLE DEMOTT: I had experience in working with people, and still I had problems in getting good aides. You are hiring someone who is not necessarily skilled or trained in the kind of care they are being asked to do, and they are probably not earning much over the minimum wage. But I discovered that if I worked with them, they were generally responsive and tried to meet our needs.

In working with an aide to get the kind of care the dying person requires, it helps considerably if the aide becomes attached and committed to the person. If the patient is alert and not in considerable pain, the caregiver can facilitate this process by telling the aide interesting and endearing things about the patient. When the person is comatose or cognitively impaired, the task is more challenging.

> PAT KNOTT: We had tapes of Lisa—audio tapes—and the nurse came, looked at Lisa's photo album, and listened to her talk and that kind of thing so that she would have more of a sense of who was inside this little body.

> ANNA KROLICK: We had pictures of my mother in the room. We wanted the aide and nurse to see what she had looked like before she got so sick and lost her hair. We also had things around that were part of her life, the family pictures, the picture of her summer home, a copy of her book, things to give a sense of who she was.

In some cases, the aide or nurse will ask for this kind of information, but if not, volunteer it.

In summary, interview the nurse or aide to determine compatibility with the patient and family. In addition, ask about the aide's training and experience with the dying person's special problems. Remember that the caregiver has a right to set limits on the aide's dress, behavior, and freedom to use the rest of the house.

Maintaining Privacy: Establishing Boundaries

One of the most difficult aspects of care which must be negotiated is the need to maintain some privacy for the dying person and family while at the same time allowing the professionals to help care. In some cases, as was noted earlier, the desire for privacy can lead people to forgo help or delay it. Depending on the space and arrangement of the home and the personalities involved, paid caregivers can either be integrated fairly smoothly or be a source of considerable uneasiness. Lucinda Klein was able to work out an arrangement that suited Joyce and herself and the nurse despite the lack of space in her apartment.

> We were supposed to have seven-day-a-week care, but we said we didn't want seven-day-a-week care—we wanted six because it was just so oppressive never being alone together. The six we kind of changed to

five and a half. The nurse would get paid for the whole sixth day but only be there a couple of hours. So we got this wonderful nurse who was coming all the time. That was nice.

It is a very strange thing to have a stranger in your life twelve hours a day. I mean, being a couple and having a third person there. It's one of those things you can't ever imagine adjusting to and then it happens and you just have to deal with it. We were pretty open with her about what was going on, about our relationship. We never came out and said we were lovers, but she had taken care of AIDS patients who were gay men and it didn't seem to be any big deal for her to be dealing with lesbians. We were ourselves around her and that was helpful. There were a couple of times when we had terrible arguments where she tried to comfort each of us and tried to help us out, which I think made us appreciate her a lot.

One of the big drawbacks we saw with Ruth, and I am sure is true of a lot of other nurses: they are in a medical setting, and what do they talk about?—they talk about other patients, talk about medical care. They talk about illness. Joyce would just go crazy sometimes just listening to hours of tales about what happened to her different relatives in the hospital and what happened to this patient and that patient. It was the last thing, having been completely abused in the hospital herself, that she needed to hear. I am sure that it is quite common because that is the common ground you have with the person, sickness.

It's hard. It would be much better to have a place for the person to get away. We were in a small apartment. It was a three-room apartment, the bedroom, the living room where Joyce's bed was, and a small kitchen with a chair and table, and Ruth would go in there and sit down sometimes.

If there are problems with professional caregivers, it is important that the caregiver come to terms with them as soon as possible either through changing personnel or establishing some boundaries concerning the behavior of the staff in the home. Discussing the problems of others with a patient is *not* considered professional behavior, and the caregiver has a perfect right to set limits on this.

As the patient approaches death, his or her physical condition deteriorates. The condition of the caregiver, too, may deteriorate as the physical and emotional strain increases. Often the need for outside help grows. Before Jim DeMott died, Lucille greatly increased the amount of care she had, both because he required it and because her own health had deteriorated to the point where she needed considerable assistance:

> The agency generally prefers that the aides work one shift, generally the same shift, so if you are also staffing multiple shifts, then you are dealing with this issue three times. If you want coverage seven days a week, you are talking five people; you are into forty-hour weeks and a lot of shifts and minimally two people for weekday and additional weekend people. With the multiple shifts, you are talking about a lot of people through your home.

Before care needs increase, the caregiver and dying person, if it is feasible, need to establish some boundaries between private family life and needs of professional caregiving. Private space will allow the family to maintain some degree of normalcy, which to some extent is the goal of a home death.

As consumers, caregivers have a right to exercise control over the services they are receiving. There is a concern that possible tensions could affect the quality of care the dying person receives. To avoid tensions, try to anticipate and deal with potential problems early. If the care an agency provides is unsatisfactory, inform the state Department of Health and the state Home Care Council or Home Care Assembly.

CHAPTER THREE

Caregiving

The Caregiver's Role

Caring for a dying person is a complex process that involves deep satisfaction, numerous frustrations, and significant responsibility. Caregivers have the satisfaction of helping the dying to retain some control over their life, to live out what is left of that life as a person (not "a patient"), and to die as dignified a death as possible. The caregiver is the key person in making this possible. The satisfaction of those who make a home death possible is immense. Their achievement, however, entails considerable difficulty and is possible only when they are willing to assume primary responsibility for what happens.

Perhaps the most vexing and difficult aspect of the care is that no matter what the caregiver does, the dying person's health, with the possibility of a few brief remissions, will continue to decline. Although the caregiver knows the person is dying, the overwhelming impulse to comfort and improve the quality of life for her or him does not diminish. The caregiver is immersed in the fight to keep the dying person eating, drinking, and taking medications, for in that direction lies life—despite the knowledge that death will come, and come soon.

In this respect, caring for someone dying at home involves a necessary denial of the impending death. It is not possible simultaneously to participate in intense caregiving and to disengage from the person in recognition of the coming death. Instead, the caregiver has to focus on what must be done each day to keep the dying person as comfortable as possible.

To say that the goal of terminal care is to keep the dying person as comfortable as possible belies this tension and incorrectly gives the impression that comfort is somehow a unified, clear, and easily achieved goal. It is not. It is very difficult to draw the line between providing comfort and artificially prolonging life, even if one excludes the use of such life-extending technology as intravenous hydration therapy (providing liquids through a needle inserted in a vein) and suctioning (removing secretions via the throat by using a suction pump). The caregiver must recognize that no matter how diligent and careful, no matter how ingenious he or she is at devising ways to nourish and medicate, there will come a time when eating, drinking, and taking medication will cease—and the person will then soon die.

This, of course, is the agreed-upon scenario when caregivers embark upon terminal care. Once the caregiver becomes committed to ongoing caregiving, however, it is difficult emotionally and psychologically to live with these contradictions. Confronting them is part of tending the dying person. The more information caregivers obtain concerning the dying process and the caregiving—whether it is from other caregivers, hospice workers, or literature such as this book—the more easily they can accept this process and their lack of responsibility for it, while at the same time maintaining the dying person's comfort.

> JOE STEAD: I was doing everything I possibly could to build her up so that she could do things, but I couldn't. I worked. I worked. I gave the best care I could give her, but it didn't work. It was really rough.

Problem Solving

Caregivers, sometimes with input from the dying person, will have the responsibility for day-to-day problem solving. Problems small and large are part of the dying process, and they are part of caring for a seriously ill person at home. Some caregivers found that accepting this responsibility and working to solve problems gave them a way of coping with the situation. It provided them with a sense of control over their lives and an important activity to preoccupy themselves with in the face of the impending death. Although these caregivers had significant professional support, they preferred to assume as much responsibility as feasible on their own.

> STAN CLARK: You concentrate on all the little symptoms and you don't look at the big picture at all. You just focus on every little thing and you

are just engrossed in that. I never put it into the big picture. Each little individual thing was responded to totally at the moment.

LUCILLE DEMOTT: There are so many things to think about. There are so many different medications, and the standard procedure calls for giving medications every six hours. So how are you going to balance that out with quality of care? You are not going to wake the person up. And remembering which medicines go with food and which do not. You literally need to work out a very complex schedule. It is completely consuming.

There will be times when something unexpected occurs and caregivers, and possibly the patient, will want to handle the problem on their own.

LUCILLE DEMOTT: It sometimes would happen when Jim was practicing walking that he would fall down in the middle of the night when no one was there but me. What do you do? Jim's approach was to call no one; the two of us could work it out ourselves. After the third time he fell, we did manage it ourselves. The first time I was in a panic. Here we had a man over six feet, weighing two hundred pounds, and me, the helper, considerably smaller. We had no lifting equipment at this time and he had very little ability to help himself.

I was so concerned, and every other woman I have heard about in this situation is so concerned, that I would never get him into "bed" that I felt a need to call someone. By the third time he fell we figured out a system to get him into bed ourselves. I just got pillows and we slept on the floor. The first time, I panicked and went to call a professional. But Jim knew we could solve the problem and he was right. If you take enough time, you can solve the problem. You need to take the time to make the situation a problem-solving one and one with a little humor.

Part of being a caregiver is accepting that incidents like this one will occur and that, in all likelihood, the caregiver and possibly the dying person can solve the problem. However, some caregivers found this level of responsibility to be a significant strain. Professional support should be available to those who want to share the responsibility. Such help is not always available, however, as Laura Sweet and Helena Wolf discovered.

HELENA WOLF: I got no support, but I didn't know enough to demand it at that point. I don't know why. I would talk to the hospice RN on the phone, but no one ever suggested any pain medicine or any medication. In retrospect, I wonder why the doctor didn't just come and give him some meds.

I finally had to call him up, and I asked if I could give Herbert some of the Valium the doctor had given me. I don't know whether it was frightening for the professionals to watch, or what. I mean, in retrospect I don't know. You are in the middle and it is very difficult to know whether what is happening to you is totally bizarre or normal. I am certainly not a retiring person, but you don't know what to be demanding for. You just sort of say, "O.K."

LAURA SWEET: There were a lot of times when I didn't know what to do. Like I didn't know how to change dressings or give a shot. Maybe we'd miss the time we were supposed to do it or something, and I wouldn't know what to do. Or, if he was feeling really bad, I didn't know if I could give him more medication or mix the medications. "Let's try this instead of that; instead of taking 6 morphines and 4 Dilaudid, let's try 12 morphines and 2 Dilaudid."

Eventually we would call a doc and find out what to do, but we got to the point when we decided they didn't know what they were doing either. We felt, "What have we got to lose?" We would try out different things. Sometimes I would call my mom, who was a nurse and had worked in a cancer hospital, and describe what was happening and she would give me advice.

Caregivers have a right to demand support for themselves in their problem solving, far more than was provided to either Laura Sweet or Helena Wolf. It may be difficult to achieve relief of pain or symptoms but the caregiver should not be alone in assuming this responsibility. In the above cases, both caregivers should have called the hospice agency or their physician and insisted on an evaluation of the care problems. If the appropriate professional is unwilling or unable to help, the caregiver should seek different professional help. Hospice agencies must have twenty-four-hour call service to be certified. If the pain is excruciating and the physician and the hospice are not available, take the person to a hospital emergency room. Such a visit will be necessary because doctors cannot order narcotic medications over the phone for patients whom they are not currently treating. If relief of pain or symptoms cannot be achieved at home, professionals need to evaluate the situation and decide whether to recommend hospitalization.

In summary, a caregiver's ability to solve problems may

give the caregiver a sense of control,
provide a needed diversion for the caregiver,
depend on the caregiver's ability to improvise,
be enhanced through professional support,
require insisting that professional support be provided,
involve locating alternate forms of professional support.

Decision Making

As death approaches and the dying person's condition deteriorates, the caregiver, with the dying person if possible, will have to decide whether or not to continue care that is increasingly difficult for the patient to endure but sustains life. Typically these decisions are characterized as "pulling the plug." But at home they are far less dramatic, occur over time, and are dictated by the person's comfort and ability to continue receiving life-sustaining care. Interventions that prolong life in the home include nourishment, prevention of infection, and medication (except pain control); usually intervention does not mean the use of life-sustaining technology, although in some cases IV hydration therapy may be considered intervention.

As an example of how difficult these decisions can be, consider the case of a cognitively impaired person (this means that the ability to think clearly is impaired by the disease process, medication, or both) who refuses to take medications necessary to sustain life, such as someone with a brain tumor who refuses to take Decadron. Does the caregiver honor the dying person's refusal to take medication or try to "sneak" the pill in? These are difficult decisions because one can never be absolutely sure, first, whether the impaired person means what he or she is saying and, second, whether stopping the medication will bring about death. In this type of situation, one must rely on one's intimate knowledge of the patient and act according to how he or she might decide if not impaired. It is important to remember in such a situation that death is already very near, and that the decision will generally affect the length of the person's life by only a few days or a week.

It is best for all concerned—the dying person, caregiver, and other relevant people such as the physician and family members—to discuss the various treatment options before the need to make decisions arises in a crisis. In many states, one can make a **living will,** which explicitly states one's wishes about what actions should be taken in the event of a medical crisis. These documents do not typically cover the often subtle decisions required in home care. However, a clear understanding of the dying person's wishes can provide general guidelines for the caregiver to follow, and, if possible, those wishes should be made clear to all the appropriate people. This can help prevent bitter conflicts among family members over treatment decisions. (Ideally, a living will should be drawn up when a person is well.)

> LUCILLE DeMOTT: I always tried to distinguish the physical changes to know where he was, but there were critical decisions like whether or not to stop the life-saving Decadron. As it turned out, I was wondering whether to withdraw the Decadron to hasten his death when he lost his swallow response. I had already called the physician to confirm a prior conversation and had said, "You told me once I could stop the Decadron to hasten Jim's death; is that accurate? Well, what will happen to him if I don't give it to him?" The doctor described the physiology and gave me very precise, detailed information starting with "From the signs you are describing, he is near death." Decision making was going on all the time. Big decisions. The life and death decisions.
>
> At the same time [as] I was struggling to make this decision, his body started shutting down. The reflex action of swallowing solids stopped a good two weeks before he died. He was eating almost nothing except milkshakes, when he could take them. When a patient is in a different stage, you might consider switching medications, but in Jim's stage you might consider whether it is worth supplying medicine at all.

In some situations the risks and benefits are relatively clear. For example, hospitals will discourage the use of **Foley catheters** because of the risk of infection, which the dying person would be too weak to fight off. However, if an **in-dwelling catheter** makes someone near death more comfortable, the risk of infection may seem trivial in comparison to the person's immediate comfort.

> ANNA KROLICK: In the hospital they taught me to do intermittent catheterization for my mother. I never got it quite right and she hated it and

found it humiliating. At one point, the hospice nurse said, "Why are we doing this?" It was clear she was going to die soon, and it was more important to me to have her comfortable than to worry about an infection, so the nurse put in a Foley catheter.

Similarly, hospitals discourage frequent enemas because they interfere with normal bowel function. But when the bowel ceases to function effectively, either through disease or as a side effect of narcotic pain medications, it may be appropriate to increase the frequency of enemas if they contribute to comfort.

Ethical Dilemmas

In preparing for a home death, the caregiver and dying person may want to consider making the following decisions in advance:

Which, if any, life-sustaining interventions should be used?
At what point, if any, should medications intended to treat the disease be discontinued?
At what point, if any, should comfort take precedence over treatment?

Deciding whether to begin or continue life-sustaining interventions to a dying person will be facilitated by a professional's assessment of how near death is. The patient is in a delicate balance; any one of a number of possible complications could cause death. Good nursing care is aimed at preventing or limiting these complications. When the dying person has six weeks or two months to live, the concern over complications is more important than when death is a few days to a week away. The closer death is, the more difficult it becomes both to administer the life-sustaining interventions and to keep the person comfortable. Choices will often have to be made between these. The choice advocated here is to do what is necessary to ensure comfort.

Although the body's gradual shutting down will frequently make the choice of discontinuing medication obvious, in the case of IV hydration therapy, the choice is less clear. When eating and drinking by mouth cease, a person cannot live longer than a few days without this therapy. There is controversy about whether IV hydration should be used at this point. Clearly, if the dying person is competent, he or she should make the decision. Hospitals tend to provide IV hydration, whereas hospices do so only if the patient or family requests it. There is uncertainty about whether more suffering is caused by dehydration or by the side effects of IV hydration. However, a consensus is building that the dying person is not made uncomfortable by the dehydration, which is part of the body's process of shutting down. Having a physician or nurse and possibly the social worker review the options and their consequences can help the dying person and family sort through the ethical and emotional issues.

Achieving comfort through the relief of pain presents an opposite problem. Here the issue is not bringing about death by stopping interventions, but the possibility of hastening death through increasing the amount of pain medication. A dying person should not have to suffer from pain. In most cases adequate pain relief should be available. If the patient is not receiving it, the caregiver should find a physician who can provide it. (See appendix B for information.) Sometimes as death approaches, pain becomes increasingly acute and more difficult to control adequately. Pain medication is then given more frequently and in larger doses.

Although physicians and nurses know what amount of pain medication constitutes a lethal dose, in particular cases this knowledge may be imprecise for two reasons. First, as the dying person takes increasingly large doses of medication to achieve control of the pain, the body builds up a tolerance. Thus someone who has built up a high tolerance for the medication may not be affected by a dose that would be lethal for someone without the tolerance. Second, as the body's functions break down in the death process, its ability to metabolize medication changes. What at one point is a safe dose may later prove to be fatal.

So, as a person dies, situations arise wherein the caregiver, physician, and nurse will not know for certain whether a dose of pain medication is lethal or not. The caregiver may be caught between the desire to control the patient's pain and the fear of accidentally ending life. Because the need for pain medication may gradually decrease as death approaches and the body's metabolism slows down, the person's pain and the amount of medication needs to be continually reevaluated. Careful evaluation by a nurse or physician will reduce the possibility of giving an accidental overdose of medication. In most cases, it is not possible to bring about death through a single inappropriate dose.

ANNA KROLICK: The last day or so before my mother died, she was in increasing pain. We kept revising how often we gave her the medication. The nurse said 50 milligrams every four hours, but that didn't seem to work. We kept calling the nurse and reducing the time and increasing the dose. Finally, whenever Elizabeth indicated she wanted more, we gave it to her.

Problems are created in the family when the dying person insists on a lethal dose of pain medication and the family opposes this wish. In such situations a reevaluation of pain control should be undertaken. Many dying people who have experienced extreme pain have a much greater fear of the pain returning than of death itself. Along with the medical and nursing evaluation, social work and possibly pastoral counseling can help to identify the source of the person's desire for medication and the family's resistance.

This is clearly a difficult, controversial area. If possible, a hospice nurse should be in the home to adjust the medications and assume responsibility for the outcome. When caregivers are alone with a patient who is in pain, they can experience a strong sense of helplessness and lack of control as a result of the dilemma they face. Relieving pain is the most urgent and crucial task of the caregiver; and the caregiver usually requires professional assistance.

Conflicts

Some of the most painful and divisive conflicts are disagreements among family members and caregivers over the way care is provided. The disagreements may concern the adequacy of pain relief, the competence of the professional staff, the decision to stop or start treatment, or who should be permitted to visit and for how long. All decisions can be extremely weighty, especially when the dying person can no longer participate competently.

There are several reasons why people may disagree with the main caregiver, or, if they share this responsibility, with the other caregivers: they may question the caregiver's competence or expertise; they may desire more control over the patient; they may be expressing guilt about lack of earlier involvement or about past actions; they may be compensating because they are afraid of death; or they may be involved in a power struggle with the caregiver over the person's care or what is to happen after death. Given the intensity of feelings, it is often difficult to resolve these problems.

The caregiver, already under extreme stress from the responsibility and physical strain of caregiving, may interpret any questioning as a lack of support or as doubts about competence, or as intrusion on an exclusive relationship such as that between husband and wife or parent and young child. In trying to resolve conflicts, the needs and the limitations of the caregivers must be balanced against the needs of the dying person. Inevitably the care the patient receives will be determined by the abilities of the primary and assisting caregivers. Dying at home creates tensions while at the same time offering opportunities for intimacy and increased contact between the caregiver and the dying person. Certified hospices have social workers on staff whose role is to help families resolve conflicts that arise in caregiving.

There are many reasons for attempting to resolve conflicts. Perhaps most immediate are the problems they cause for the dying person: emotional and even physical suffering. Research has shown (Melzack 1990) that people experiencing emotional distress are less able to tolerate pain than those who are calm. A calm environment, then, will help the patient tolerate pain and will give him or her the satisfaction of leaving a family at peace rather than in conflict. This calm will also allow the person to turn attention inward and prepare for death.

Most immediately, conflicts significantly impair the caregiver's ability to give safe and competent care. Some conflicts clearly concern the well-being and needs of the family members. Family members want to settle accounts or to have reconciliations. Both the dying person and those who will live on have needs that must be considered. But conflicts also impede the caregiver's ability to come to terms with the dying person. It is important to remember that death is irrevocable, final—there is no "later" chance for resolution. Resolving conflicts (or controlling them, if resolution is not possible) will help the caregivers to take their leave of the dying person.

HELENA WOLF: My brothers and father were estranged, which made life difficult. When it became clear that Herbert was quite sick, I called my brother Ron, whom he had not talked to in five years. I also had not talked to Ron. I just called him up. Ron was concerned but aloof. We then began to interact. Ron would call me. I would call him. My other brother Sam, with whom he was in contact, was away on vacation. I eventually called Sam on vacation and we got into the habit of talking every day. My brother Ron sent Father some flowers, which he dismissed. Herbert would have nothing to do with deathbed reconciliations. Ron and Sam both wanted to come and see Herbert when he was still here. I told Herbert that I told them, and he was very angry at me, [said] that was none of my business, that he didn't want people to know he was sick. Eventually, Herbert made this incredible scene: they might come but he wouldn't see them. There would be no deathbed reconciliations. Whatever was going to be worked out had to have been worked out before. The fact that he was dying had nothing to do with this.

Herbert refused to see them. He made my husband call them and tell them not to come. In retrospect, did we do the right thing? Herbert was certainly adamant; we certainly did what he wanted, but was that really what he wanted? Should he have been second-guessed? I don't know. I mean, we tried. He appeared totally competent at the time. There was no question that that was what he wanted; he didn't want to see them. Ron and Sam both came right away after Herbert went into the hospital. At that point he was totally out of it and didn't know they were there.

Conflicts in which the needs of the living must be balanced against those of the dying are extremely difficult to resolve. In some cases it may be appropriate to have a mental health professional assess the situation. In cases like Helena Wolf's, where events happened quickly, it is important to ascertain whether the person fully comprehends that he or she is dying. Such an evaluation can help in making decisions, but only those close to the dying person can assess the impact of trying to resolve a conflict. Although the tendency in the cases discussed here was to honor the wishes of the patient, it is those who live on who will have to come to terms with the results of the decisions.

With remarriages, resolution is often difficult, especially when the person dying has a second family and animosity from the divorce is carried over into the caregiving. When hospitals face these kinds of conflicts, they resolve them by strictly alternating the periods when each family can visit the patient. But at home there is no neutral structure to impose a system for dealing with the conflict, which may not be resolved, even though the person is dying. At home the antagonistic families must deal with each other, perhaps for the first time. Lucille DeMott and the adult children of Jim's first marriage who had come to town to help care for their father tried to resolve their antagonisms but ultimately failed:

> If I had it to do over again, I would have said no visitors, as he became more ill and less responsive, that it was not appropriate to be with him more than fifteen minutes at a time or more than once or twice a day. But I was not smart enough to do that. I vacillated. Jim would tell me that he didn't want people there. He wouldn't tell them that, of course. At first I would suggest coming later in the day. Then I would tell them —these were people who did not have a high regard for me—"He really needs a shorter time span."
>
> But then they wouldn't want to leave, which is understandable. So I said, "How about one person in the room at a time and the rest of you stay downstairs and give him some rest?" I tried all kind of things. When it really came to a head one day was when the father and the sister and the two kids and the spouse of one of the kids had been up in either the bedroom or doorway for a while and Jim was totally nonresponsive. My original philosophy was that that was O.K. They should be there and participate in the caring. So there was a part of me that thought that this was the way it ought to be, but Jim had told me he didn't want anyone but me involved in intimate care. I went upstairs and found him with the covers off and partially nude, which of course he would never have wanted. His dignity was of the most importance to him.
>
> I covered him up and went downstairs still not knowing what to do. It was a terrible dilemma. I finally just went upstairs and asked them to leave. The family came downstairs and I told them, "I can't let you visit with him so long with so many people anymore. I have tried every way to let you know that the length of visits are too much for him, too many people are too much for him, so we aren't going to do this anymore." Then I was seen as the villain. There seemed to be no way to satisfy everyone's needs.

Longstanding family conflicts, which may affect caregiving, take on a special urgency because one of the main actors is soon to die and the conflicts may never be resolved. The people involved must try to work things out. In some situations, talking may not be sufficient or even possible. This is what Lucille DeMott found out:

The family refused to talk with me, so I am not sure what could have prevented the conflict. We were in a conflictful situation among relatives, all of whom loved him and cared for him. Whatever one could do to sit down and discuss feelings, processes, and visits earlier would have been very, very useful.

When we talked to each other, we tended to discuss the death and the cancer process and which music and movies he would like to see, but not the critical issue to them, which was money. I didn't realize that was the issue. Part of what was creating all the trouble over visits was that the issue that was very important to them was not known to me at the time.

One way for caregivers to communicate that families have found helpful, as well as a good method for organizing caregiving, is **family rounds.** This is simply a time each day when those involved in the actual caregiving set aside a period, possibly a meal, when they can all be present and discuss the care of the dying person, problems they are having, and their individual assessments of what is happening. And they find solutions. A friend or neighbor can play an invaluable role here by sitting with the patient so that all the caregivers can meet. This is also a good opportunity to identify conflicts. However, there might not be the time or the calm to resolve the conflict. If more work is needed, it might be possible to meet in a neutral setting, such as the hospice office.

Many informants expressed the wish that some neutral party had been there who could have helped them resolve the conflicts that inevitably arose.

HELENA WOLF: Dealing with [family] conflicts is the kind of thing which you never think about when you decide to have someone at home. Maybe if he had been in a hospital or nursing home there would have been someone else there, a social worker to run the ramparts, and maybe he would have dealt with some of this [conflict] on his own.

Hospitals and nursing homes often do not provide this kind of professional help. Hospices, however, are committed to helping the family deal with the death. Their philosophy is that family conflicts must be resolved, or at least eased, to free the family members to provide emotional support for the dying person and to create a peaceful atmosphere in which to die. Hospices that are certified must have a social worker who is available to help families resolve these situations. If conflict is expected, using a certified hospice agency should be considered.

The decision to use professional help in resolving family conflicts can relieve the caregiver and other family members of the additional strain. For the caregiver, the task diverts energy better spent on the dying person.

> LAURA SWEET: I was really timid about asking for help. It is partly the way I was brought up. I should have asked for more help from Anthony's family directly. They always said, "Let us know if you need any help." But it is hard to ask. You can't.

In resolving conflicts, the following means may be helpful:

- Consult a social worker, psychologist, or psychiatrist who has experience in resolving interpersonal conflicts.
- Consider the importance of finding solutions for the dying person's well-being and peace of mind.
- If necessary, alternate periods of visiting for family members or friends who cannot resolve their conflict.
- If necessary, set limits on how long and how often visitors may visit the patient.
- Schedule family rounds, when all caregivers and family members meet to discuss problems and work on finding solutions. (See chapter 7 for discussion of practical concerns that may require group participation.)

The Dignity and Autonomy of the Dying Person

A key aspect of home death is the caregiver's ability to provide the dying person with dignity through this last period of life.

> LUCILLE DeMOTT: Throughout all this we fought for dignity and respect for the patient. That to me still was the main thing. Protecting the dignity of the patient—maintaining the patient's rights in the same way as if he were not a patient. If the patient likes privacy, you give him privacy.

> STAN CLARK: The nurse was really amazing in her sensitivity to Alice. She never came up to her and just threw the covers off like a lot of

hospital nurses did. Instead, she was always very careful to keep Alice covered and to preserve her dignity.

Dignity means protecting the person's personal modesty, integrity, and right to make decisions about his or her own life. It is this last aspect—the ability to exercise control—which is most closely tied to adult identity in our culture in the United States. Relinquishing that prerogative is equivalent to losing an adult identity; it is a kind of social death. It is important, therefore, to allow the dying to exercise control over as much of their lives as possible.

Individuals facing death sometimes feel they have completely lost control of their lives. It is all too easy for a caregiver to assume more decision-making power than is warranted by the patient's condition. To guard against this, it is often possible to work with the dying person to establish a kind of shared autonomy; that is, the patient delegates decision-making responsibility to the caregiver. In so doing, the dying person retains the authority to delegate a responsibility. This can be done legally by assigning the caregiver or someone else legal power of attorney.

Whenever possible, the dying person should be involved in decision making. Even when cognitive impairment is present, it is rarely total. Careful assessment can often identify areas where the person remains competent and is able to participate. Presenting information and choices in terms that are easy to understand helps the dying person participate.

Having a daily routine that the dying person helps establish will give some sense of control over life. Asking what food the person wants, which visitors should come, when various procedures should be done, and who should be present all help enhance sense of control over life and hence personal dignity.

There comes a time in the disease and dying process when the dying person is barely able to make decisions, when control must be relinquished. In situations where the patient is competent, he or she must negotiate with the caregiver these boundaries of personal integrity and control and the changes that will take place as the person withdraws from society. In some cases, it is very difficult for the caregiver to move in and assume control as the person withdraws. This typically happens when roles are reversed, as when a wife assumes control of a previously dominant husband, or a child of a parent. In such cases, serious problems can develop when the caregiver continues to rely on the dying person long after he or she is unable to make decisions. When a serious gap in authority occurs, hospice personnel may assume responsibility, but they do this reluctantly. If the dying person's safety is threatened, however, the hospice will become more involved.

Becoming an Expert

Caring for the terminally ill is not simply a matter of fluffing pillows and making chicken soup. Although performing much of the medical care necessary to extend life is unnecessary, intense nursing care is usually required (see appendix A for information on nursing care): such things as getting the person to eat and drink in sufficient amounts to keep living, persuading the patient to take medication, controlling pain, attending to skin care and hygiene, and numerous other tasks. In many cases, maintaining the dying person's comfort can be an immensely demanding, complex task; yet these demands must be balanced against the other goal of home death—allowing the dying person to live out the remainder of life with dignity at home.

It is the role of the professionals to assist and guide the caregiver in this task. Unless they are there twenty-four hours a day, however, they will rely on the caregiver to help identify problems and evaluate the success of various solutions as well as to provide most of the nursing care. The caregiver assumes the role of expert on the patient. This is also a key role the caregiver can play for a hospitalized patient.

The Patient Log

The dying person, when lucid and willing to think about care problems, can help the caregiver collect and analyze the information that the physician or nurse needs. But the patient may not be sufficiently lucid or may not want to participate, in which case the caregiver assumes responsibility for the observations. It helps to keep a **patient log** and pill schedule (see figure 1 on pages 96–97), which record medication, nourishment, and care problems.

If the dying person is able to help, keeping the log represents a significant part of the control that he or she can exercise over life. The log should include information on the onset of pain, the time and amount of medication taken, and the time it takes for the medication to take effect (that is, relief of pain, sleep, or calmness). A hardback stenographer's notebook is ideal for this purpose.

The log can contain information vital to continued effective care. When pain medications are used, it is essential to keep a careful record of the amount and time of each dose. The physician or hospice nurse will need to know how much the patient is getting in order to monitor its effect on the body, including how well it controls pain. The log is also an important reminder of when and how much medication has been given. This is key when more than one caregiver is involved and as caregivers themselves become progressively run-down and less able to recall clearly when and how much medication was given.

The log should be kept by the patient's bed, and an entry should be made each time medication is given and a meal is taken. Any special circumstances should be noted. Additional observations pertaining to the dying person's condition should be included if time permits.

Maintaining the log can help the caregiver and the dying person organize their information and observations and present them to the physician or nurse in a fashion that will make it easier for them to assess the situation. After the person dies, the log will serve the caregiver and family members as a record of these last days. In the intensity and exhaustion of caregiving, it is not at all easy to remember the details—details that at the time seemed etched forever on the participants' minds.

PAT KNOTT: I had lots of decisions to make at that point about Lisa and how much she was vomiting and did we need to cut back on the richness of her liquid food. There were all kinds of routine decisions that were being made as she went through different kinds of chemo. Was this reaction more than it should have been to this med? Should I call someone? We kept a little log so that we could keep track of what was happening. When Don would come, he would ask me how the day had gone and pick up the log, which we kept at the foot of the bed and look at how many times she had been ill or how the diarrhea was doing and how her skin was holding up.

The log's usefulness may be limited in some cases. Caregivers can put considerable effort into meticulously maintaining the log,

March 31, April 1 + 2

		Thursday 3/31		Friday 4/1		Saturday 4/2	
		Time + Dose	Condition	Time + Dose	Condition	Time + Dose	Condition
4 AM – 6 AM	Injection Surfak #1	4:00 (.8)	no pain, joint stiffness, sore fingers	5:00 (8cc)	sleepy, fed, enema	3:30 .8 cc / 3:30 2 valium	
7 AM – 9 AM	dolophine Theodore Valium	2 7AM / 1 " / 1 "	no pain, mild joint stiffness, hiccoughs	2 8AM / 1 " / 1 "	9:00 suppository 9:30 BM	2 / 1 / 1	9 AM radiation appt.
10 AM – noon	MD Inject Surfak (#2) Valium 1½ hrs after feeling aggression, dull pain in side	.5cc / 1 11:00 / 1 11:00 / 1 12:30	after 5 min, unusual response, cramps + decrease fluid in head	12:30	11:00 radiation appt.		
1 PM – 3 PM	Dolophine Theodur E mcgt (#2) Valium	1 1:50 / 1 3:10 / 1 / 1	sleeps, alert, little bit groggy, pain	2:30 6mg / 3:00 / 1 " / 10 mg 1:00	general float		
4 PM to 6 PM	MS Inject Surfak #3 Valium	10mg MS / 1 (4:30) / 1 (4:30) Val. 6:30 pm	vomiting, bad cramps	5:45 .4cc / 4 PM / 2 6:30	good urination, slow melon + milk		
7 PM – 9 PM	Dolophine Theodur Emcgt #3 Valium	2 8:00 / 1 " / 1 " / 7:00 / 8:30 (dig)	Build up of pain, discomfort	4PM / 4PM / 4PM / 8:30 m.s.	8:50 pm Val IV		
10 pm – midnight	MS Inject Elavil 75 mg Surfak #4	.8cc / 1 (10:45) / 1 (10:45)	Δ pain	10:30 MS / 1 12:00			
1 AM – 3 AM	Dolophine Theodur	2 val. 2 AM / 2 Dol. 2 AM / 1 Theo.					

Figure 1. Patient Log (above) and Pill Schedule (right)

Jim's pill schedule, Sat., March 6 - Friday, March 11
2 percocet every 3 hours, and Dalmane at night
(Warm books and heating pad gave relief - slept nights.
Radiation Wed. - Sat.

		Sat 3-5	Sun 3-6	Mon 3-7	Tues 3-8	Wed 3-9	Thurs 3-10	Friday 3-11
5 AM	2 percocet	✓	✓	✓	✓	✓	✓	✓
	stool softener	✓	✓	✓	✓	✓	✓	✓
	compazine					(c)✓		
8 AM	1 dolophine	✓	✓	✓	✓	✓	✓	✓
	1 Theodor	✓	✓	✓	✓	✓	✓	✓
	valium compazine				(v)9:30	(v)9:30 (c)10:00		
11 AM	2 percocet / stool softener	✓	✓	✓	✓	✓	✓	✓
	valium compazine elavil						((c)25)	(c)1:15
2 PM	1 dolophine	2tab ✓	✓	✓	✓			
	1 Theodor	✓	✓	✓	✓			
5 PM	2 percocet	✓	✓	✓	✓	✓	✓	✓
	1 stool softener	✓	✓	✓	✓	✓	✓	✓
	6:00 compazine			✓	✓	✓	✓	
8 PM	1 dolophine	✓	✓	✓	✓	✓	✓	
	1 Theodor	✓	✓		✓	✓	✓	
	compazine elavil			(c)10:00	(c)9:00 (s)25mg			
11 PM	2 percocet	✓	✓	✓		✓	✓	✓
	1 elavil (75 mg)	✓	✓			✓	✓	✓
	Sleeping well at night							
2 AM	1 dolophine	2tab ✓	✓		✓	✓	✓	
	1 Theodor	✓	✓		✓	✓	✓	
Wed.	After radiation, intense pain + weakness in thighs							
Thurs	felt better today							
Sat.	2 games Trivial Pursuit							

only to be disappointed if relief of pain or symptoms is still elusive.* Relief of symptoms is difficult to achieve when there is an inadequate scientific understanding of the disease and the dying process. It is usually not the caregiver's information that is responsible. The log remains a valuable aspect of safe and effective caregiving, but it may not provide the solution to all caregiving problems.

Figure 1 is an excerpt from a patient's log and one week of his pill schedule. In making up a log, be sure to leave ample space for comments about the kinds of problems encountered; the location, intensity, and quality of pain; and the effectiveness of a particular drug in combating the problem.

The Quality of Life

Having someone die at home often gives care and attention unobtainable in an institutional setting and allows the person to live as normal a life as possible. Maintaining something like a normal family life can be a major achievement if the patient is very sick and debilitated. It can also be a major source of satisfaction. Every attempt should be made to provide the things that the person enjoyed while in good health. Experiencing these, even in a limited fashion, will have a pleasurable association and invoke positive memories of good times past.

> LUCILLE DeMOTT: We had lots of parties while Jim was ill: we just moved the parties up into the bedroom. People came up and we had cocktails and dinner and had kids' birthday parties. There was a lot of celebration going on. This was not only a down-in-the-mouth time, a tragic time. You know you have to live your life; you just live it in that room.

Life, of course, is not normal, and the dying person is confined to the home, often to one room. Two of the terminally ill in this study were able to continue their work in a limited fashion until days before their deaths. For others this was impossible, and they faced long periods of potentially empty time. Although the dying may sleep for considerable portions of the day, there are times when they need social interaction and diversion. The most satisfying kinds of

---

* If the physician or nurse fails to relieve the pain and makes no use of the patient log, consider switching to a different doctor or nurse.

diversions are those which have some meaning for the caregiver as well as the dying person.

> HELENA WOLF: It was all stressful but it wasn't absolutely unhappy. Once I said "O.K., Dad, you have to tell me your recipe for chicken paprikas." So we had this great conversation and he told me the different things he knew how to make. Then we looked through some old family photos and he told me who everyone was.

The caregiver and patient may enjoy sharing some of these diversions:

- Watching home videos
- Listening to music
- Looking through family picture albums
- Going outside (The feel of fresh air is especially valued by people usually confined indoors.)
- Smelling and applying different lotions and creams (Because the sense of smell is so acute and one of the last to go, dying people can enjoy the sensuous nature of fragrant creams or powders or aromatic scents when other sensuous pleasures such as eating are lost to them.)
- Maintaining a ritual of drinking tea or a cocktail at a specific time of day (This gives a person something to look forward to and breaks the monotony of a caregiving routine.)

One of the more satisfying achievements for the caregiver and dying person is to invent ways to surmount the limitations created by weakness and disease. Even a simple excursion out of doors can be a major achievement for the caregiver and a source of enjoyment for the patient.

> ANNA KROLICK: There was one beautiful, warm fall day and we decided we had to get my mother out to see it. My brother-in-law and I made a bed out of concrete blocks and pieces of foam rubber which was high enough to transfer her and then rigged up a blanket between two ladders to give her some shade. Then he picked her up and carried her outside. We put some flowers near her face, and my stepdaughter had her puppy play nearby to keep our kids playing around Mother's bed. It was a wonderful scene.

Caring for someone dying at home is an extremely complex and demanding process. Caregivers do not need advanced training or professional know-how. They do need physical and emotional stamina, a willingness to learn, and the ability to assume significant responsibilities. Professional support should make the caregiver's job easier. Professionals provide the caregiver with training, information, reassurance, and collaboration in decision making, as well as hands-on care. If caregivers are not receiving this kind of support, they should consider changing agencies. Despite the difficulties, helping someone die at home allows the caregiver to maximize the positive aspects of the patient's last days and to ensure that the care that is provided fits the needs, desires, and beliefs of the dying person.

CHAPTER FOUR

Social Support

I believe that this is the time for celebration, for a lot of people to be there. I don't see the death process as a one-on-one relationship time.

—Lucille DeMott

It was something I felt I just had to do if I was going to be part of this community.

—A friend who helped care for Elizabeth Krolick

In conducting the research for this book, I was consistently struck by the significance that caregivers attached to the contributions of others, both positive and negative. Years after a death, caregivers vividly recounted small gestures that had made a deep impression on them. They equally vividly described, with considerable pain, incidents when expected signs of support had not materialized. Some of those who provided the support said it was one of the most meaningful things they had done in their lives. This chapter describes the role the informal support system plays in the care of a person dying at home. It examines the tensions and anguish created when social support is inadequate or not forthcoming. It will offer some explanations for the extreme significance attached to support during this crisis period. It discusses one of the most difficult aspects of caregiving: the emotional conflicts that inevitably occur. In such a highly charged, emotional atmosphere as tending a dying family member, conflicts among the caregivers are likely, especially if there are serious problems predating the terminal illness. The chapter ends with a discussion of the role of children in caring for the dying.

This chapter is written for those who wish to provide support for the main caregiver or caregivers. It addresses those people who wish in some way to help and to demonstrate their caring and commitment to either the dying person or the caregiver or both. Included in this group are less intimate friends, colleagues, and neighbors, as well as the friends and family members who come to play a significant and essential supportive role in the care of the dying. Caregivers too may wish to read this chapter for assistance in understanding how social support can work and why it is so important.

The Meaning of Social Support

All of the informants in this book made the decision to care for the dying person at home with the expectation that family and friends would help, an involvement that the hospice philosophy explicitly promotes. In contrast to the hospital, where death is seen as a medical event, hospice defines death socially. It is concerned with the dying person as a *whole* person, with social, emotional, and psychological needs, and as a person who is meaningfully connected to other people. The dying process is one of disengagement from these social ties. The medical and nursing interventions that hospice uses are designed to control pain and symptoms so that the patient can focus on coming to terms with death and saying good-bye to loved ones. Several caregivers approached their task with this philosophy very much in mind.

> LUCILLE DeMOTT: I had a kind of hospice view that you ought to be surrounded by the people you love and have access to them. It ought to be really quite open.

> STAN CLARK: We were very sociable; we had a lot of friends; our house was a very comfortable place for people to come. My wife liked to drink and was always a sociable person in that way—she was always ready to have fun. So our friends came over when she was dying. There was no isolation that I can remember.

Social support can take many different forms, from gestures showing one cares to **instrumental support** that may involve actually helping with the caregiving. Instrumental support refers to assistance to the caregiver. Such help can include providing meals, transportation, child care, and sitting with the dying person. The variety of supportive actions is nearly limitless, bounded only by imagination and sensitivity. Support by family members is essential to effective caregiving and to the caregiver's ability to carry on. Family members can actually relieve and substitute for the main caregiver in providing hands-on care in some cases. Only under certain circumstances (which will be discussed) can friends perform this role.

Social support also serves as an expression of other people's concern about and commitment to the caregiver and the dying person. In this sense it can act as the affirmation of friendship and affection. Conversely, if it is absent, it can bring the stability or even existence of the relationship into question. For this reason, support during a crisis such as the care of a dying family member assumes significance far beyond the nourishment contained in the chicken soup brought to the home or the phone call not made. Thus social support plays a double role in caregiving. It supplies needed, even essential, instrumental assistance to the caregiver and sometimes the patient; and it symbolizes the care and concern of the wider social group. Its presence is keenly valued and its absence acutely felt.

> PAT KNOTT: Things happen to friendships in these situations. We had a couple of friends that we had been friends with for years. They had a child a year older than Lisa, and I am certain because of their grief, because they were very attached to her, they just stopped calling and coming around. Even though we keep in touch with them, it profoundly changed the relationship. There were these other people who we knew but didn't know very well who for some reason were able to reach out and help us.

> BONNIE STEINER: We had very little family support and this is something I am just resolving now with my sister [five years later].

> HELEN WRIGHT: The fact that I would call the children and they would call me was a support constantly, and people from church, and my knowledge that they were there being supportive, writing letters.

Types of Support

Support is usually focused on either the dying person or the caregiver—though sometimes on both. Much of the support for the dying person consists of symbolic acts that attest to the affection and commitment a person feels for the one who is dying. This support is distinctly different from the hands-on caring of the caregiver and from the instrumental and emotional support of others for the caregiver.

Much of the support provided by non–family members is aimed at the caregiver, for several reasons. As the caregiver focuses on the increasingly intense demands and needs of the dying person, the support network can move in to care for the caregiver. By relieving the caregiver of adult responsibilities, such as shopping, food preparation, child care, transportation, housecleaning, and in some cases some professional responsibilities, the support network allows the caregiver to care for the dying person.

Support for the Dying Person

Except in rare cases, support focused on the dying person by non–family members is primarily spiritual and emotional. Friends and colleagues can visit and sit by the patient, send cards, letters, or gifts, or call. Letters, tapes, or videotapes in some cases, offer a particular advantage for communicating with the dying person because he or she can read or listen to them and appreciate the feelings of the sender without having to expend the effort necessary to communicate with another. Letters and audio- and videotapes also have the advantage that, for many people, it is easier to express deep feelings when the recipient is not present.

The support visits by friends or colleagues can help the dying to retain a sense of self, however briefly, for it allows them to present a more normal, intact face to the world.

> HELENA WOLF: Herbert liked the way my husband made soft-boiled eggs better than [mine]. Herbert could be gracious with him and appreciative of things he was doing for him at a time when I did the same things and I got criticized. He gave Herbert a sense of public, and he would put on a public face when he was around.

> ANNA KROLICK: We were very moved by the visits of the college kids from the place where Mother had worked. She would pull herself together and ask them about themselves and about the store. But she could only do it for a little while and the effort exhausted her.

Visits by those who provide this kind of support should be limited in time and be prearranged. It requires effort for a dying person to organize a public face, to respond appropriately to a social exchange. It also requires effort for the caregiver to behave in a socially appropriate manner, observing the kinds of conventions that are expected when adults visit each other.

The help of a neutral person who functions as a gatekeeper can be extremely important in both protecting the energy and privacy of the family and preserving relationships that must continue after the person is dead. In Alice Clark's office, the administrative assistant took it upon herself to organize the visits by colleagues to the Clarks' home. She scheduled people in groups of three with only one group a day visiting. She kept in close touch with the family to make sure that Alice was able to receive visitors that day and would cancel and reschedule visits when she wasn't. This person was able to direct people the Clarks didn't wish to see into other forms of expressing their feelings about them.

People outside the family rarely help with actual hands-on care. Hands-on care means feedings, medication, turning, assisting in movement. Even within families there are differences as to who can provide intimate hands-on care. Some families make distinctions between what a spouse can do and what adult children can do. In others, one or two people become responsible for hands-on care. Rarely is it shared by all caregivers. If the dying person is alert, he or she should be consulted about who should perform this kind of care. Sometimes the patient prefers that a paid attendant or nurse do it. In part this may be because the professional is more competent, but, significantly, it may help some people to preserve their dignity if intimate care is performed by strangers who have a professional distance.

LUCILLE DeMOTT: His adult children were integrated into the support system by selecting the music and videotapes and reading to him but doing no personal care, for the simple reason of maintaining Jim's dignity. This was a man who kissed only his wife on the lips; he didn't kiss his children on the lips. He had very explicit standards about what he thought was appropriate and inappropriate outside of a husband-and-wife relationship.

FLORENCE MARTIN: He threw a fit when I left for a day and his adult sons took care of him. He was a very proud man, and to have to have your sons unzip your pants so you can go to the bathroom was humiliating. He blamed me that his sons would see this, but I had to get away. I could understand his feelings, but I had to survive.

In some cases informal support can be used in actual hands-on care, but this is usually under specific circumstances. The people who provide this care usually have professional expertise or experience in caring for someone dying at home. People who assist in this way should have some prior experience. This is a considerable responsibility, and often people who wish to help have no idea of how seriously sick a dying person is and how much care they require. Caring for a terminally ill patient is not like coming to sit with a sick friend. For example, the common assumption that the dying person, if an adult, is capable of remaining alone for a while if the outside person is late is totally wrong in most cases. People who help in this way *must* understand the vulnerability and dependence of the dying person. Unfortunately, Anthony Lane's family did not understand this.

LAURA SWEET: At one point I had to go away on a business trip to New York, and I told his family that I was leaving here Friday and needed someone here Friday to take him to their home and bring him back Tuesday. I called Friday night—I don't know why—I just called the apartment just to find out if he was there, and he was there. I said, "Didn't anyone come down to get you?" and he was crying because he was in pain and he was alone, and I felt horrible. Here I was in New York at a trade show of all things, and I wouldn't have gone if I thought that no one was going to take care of him.

Support for the Caregiver

Most people outside the family who contribute active, instrumental support have a relationship with the caregiver. People give support in part because they observe that their friend or colleague needs help; and in part they do so because they wish to affirm their friendship for the caregiver. Modern American society does not offer many opportunities for people to express in a significant and intimate way the depth of their feelings for a friend. The usual social occasions such as dinners, picnics, parties, and sporting events rarely offer such opportunities. Helping a friend in need presents such an opportunity. These small gestures of support symbolize the friendship and affection that underlie them, and they are vividly remembered years later.

ANNA KROLICK: I remember when Elizabeth came home she desperately wanted a drink of some special brandy. I knew this friend of ours had some and called and asked him if I could come out and get some. He offered to bring it, and both he and his wife drove across town. The significance of what they did was not lost on me.

STAN CLARK: I was complaining once that I would like to have a phone by Alice's bed and one colleague said, "My son will come over tomorrow and do it." He just came over and installed the phone. They didn't have the right phone pieces and he had to go here or there, but they just did that without any disruption to us. It was so helpful.

HELENA WOLF: My friend Else came when Herbert had to go to the hospital and drove us to the hospital. It doesn't seem like a big thing, but I didn't have to think about where to park the car. That kind of thing, those kinds of things, [are] seemingly very little but in fact very helpful.

LAURA SWEET: Once a friend from work called me and said, "Can I come over and borrow your laundry?" It was so nice of her—the thought that she would drive all the way out here and pick up my laundry really touched me.

Many people who are involved with the dying person and caregiver live too far away to participate in the actual instrumental support. They can still make an invaluable contribution, however, by keeping in touch and letting both know they are thinking of them.

HELEN WRIGHT: One of the things I think I did real well was to call people up and let them know if he wanted visits and to get postcards out to all the people we knew everywhere, to let them know how he was so they could write. So there were lots and lots of letters for months and months and months—lots of appreciation. Lots of calls. I would make lots of calls, long distance to people all over the country. They would call me. I spent a lot of time on the phone being sort of a bridge so they could send their energy and pray, and so I felt that that was a very wonderful experience, and he felt so, too, to have that wide network of support. I think I really did a good job and felt really good about taking the time to keep in touch with people who wanted to know.

PAT KNOTT: I have a brother whom I am particularly close to. He wasn't able to be there but he would write short notes, and usually they would be sort of upbeat and he has a really funny sense of humor. I always found them refreshing because I was able to smile for a little.

When the caregiver initiates phone contacts, they can serve as an important source of social contact which the caregiver can control and which don't require preparation. Incoming calls, however, can become a burden. People want to help and to show their support. Telling each caller the dying person's status, answering their questions, responding to their emotional needs, can end up being more stressful than helpful. Helena Wolf found this especially difficult and solved the problem by using an answering machine:

We put an answering machine on the phone, regardless even when we were home. The telephone becomes this terrible intrusion; you want people to call but you know that it is going to be an intrusion; yet you don't know how else to be in touch with people. The phone machine allows you to moderate. Then at least people feel they can be in touch and you feel you can be in control. What happens is, people call up and sort of say, "Did he die yet?" What are you supposed to say? "Well, not yet, call back tomorrow." But you understand what they want but it's still incredibly hard. So [a] simple thing like the answering machine was a wonderful mediator.

Spiritual Support

Spiritual support can be an important role for the informal support network in addition to that provided by hospice and the clergy. The dying person can be immensely comforted by the knowledge of the prayers of others. Many caregivers, whether religious or not, are moved by the concern and love for the dying person which the prayers and devotions represent.

HELEN WRIGHT: The members of our church and the healing they performed and all those who had more of a spiritual approach were really helpful to him and to me.

MARY ROEHM: The Father was always available when I needed to talk. He was so helpful, and one of the sisters visited us regularly.

ANNA KROLICK: I'm not very religious, but when people called up and said they were praying for us, I was very moved by the thought of how intensely they were connected to us and to what was happening. And I knew my mother liked it.

In offering spiritual support, however, ascertain whether the dying person or caregiver wants it. Although religion is a great source of strength for many at a time like this, sometimes caregivers and patients see spiritual support, especially when it is provided in place of expected practical support, as demonstrating a lack of appreciation for how extremely difficult their situation is. Caregivers especially may feel this way.

LAURA SWEET: His parents were very religious. They were very good about sending cards twice a week with religious sayings. But Anthony would throw them across the room. They didn't help us. We prayed every night. We would have loved a miracle but it didn't work. I think they were just hiding behind "It's in God's hands." But it wasn't. I felt that it was in my hands and Anthony's hands.

Of course, one can respect such wishes and feelings of the patient and caregiver and still offer prayers privately in their support.

It is important to remember in such situations that if the caregiver believes that the person offering spiritual support does not understand what the caregiver is going through, the offer can have the unintended effect of making the caregiver feel misunderstood rather than comforted.

PAT KNOTT: I grew very tired of people saying that the strong can handle these kinds of things, and I used to think, "Let me be weak, then. I don't want to be strong if this is what I am supposed to handle." So many times I heard it that I remember one time just holding it inside because I just wanted to scream at this person because it was just one time too many. It was not a helpful comment. I think it is embedded in religious beliefs. It seemed to be something that a lot of people have learned to fall back on.

Caregivers who are faced with unwanted and intrusive spiritual support of the kind discussed above can make a practice of ventilating their feelings to someone else. This will prevent a buildup of irritation and allow the caregiver to deal with the next such episode.

Inevitably, people will offer spiritual support to the caregiver, and those who do not welcome it need to find a way to deal with this without letting it become disruptive.

How the Support System Works

Decision Making

Support from friends and relatives is essential to the caregiver's ability to continue to care for the dying person at home. Yet often, to identify their needs and the means by which they can be met represents an additional strain for the caregiver already preoccupied and burdened by the demands of caregiving. The most successful support is based on the willingness and ability of people simply to decide what they are going to do for the caregiver *to help with day-to-day tasks* and then to do it. Yet in many ways, it is the most difficult course to take, for it is an intrusion into the autonomy of another adult and family. In our culture this is appropriate only for behavior toward children, and even then it may be questioned. However, most caregivers in this study appreciated it when those providing assistance simply decided what they would do and did it, thus relieving them of one more decision.

PAT KNOTT: The church group got really frustrated because we kept saying, "We are all right. We will handle it." They finally had a special meeting and talked about their plan of attack and they came to us and said, "This is the way it is going to be: we are bringing you meals three times a week." The meals were generally large enough that you ate them the whole week. "And you are going to give us your schedule of chemo and someone will be here to drive you every single time." A little later on as they watched us wear down, they said, "Someone is coming for an hour and a half every morning and you are doing something; you are not staying here." They just sort of did it; they said we are going to do these things.

Many of them said afterwards that once they got to the point of telling us what they were going to do, they felt better. Before they had felt so useless and helpless. When they had asked me what they could do to help, I would just say, "Well, I don't know." I was just—you just don't think clearly. You are really overwhelmed so if somebody takes some part of what your overall responsibility is and relieves you of it, whatever it is seems like a relief because it is just one more thing that you don't have to think about and do.

It is hard to make decisions because of how exhausted you are and because of how grieved you are, and if somebody makes a decision and tells you how they are going to help you, you'll take it even if normally you wouldn't think of having somebody decide for you.

LUCILLE DeMOTT: It was one of those things where people would ask what they could do. One mother just decided to handle child care and called up three other mothers and organized something for our son. I could have set that up if I had thought of it. But it really helped that she did that.

ANNA KROLICK: Sometimes friends would call up and say, "How many people are in the house tonight for dinner?" and just cook for us all. I really appreciated not having to go through all that "Oh, you don't have to" stuff when I really needed the help and they of course knew it. After a while I could just tell people how to help when they called. My husband had a hard time with it, though, and kept wanting me to make lists of all the people who had helped so we could pay them back in some way.

It is important to note here that this is not the recommended style of making decisions regarding primary caregiving responsibilities and tasks. In these cases, decisions need to take into account the needs and perceptions of the dying person as well as the different primary caregivers. (See chapter 3 for a detailed discussion for potential problems in decision making.) The people immediately involved and family members who cannot be present usually want to participate in the decisions regarding actual care. In fact, it is precisely because there are so many decisions to be made that caregivers welcome the release from deciding about day-to-day activities and problems.

Integrating Support into the Caregiving Routine

In some cases, the support system becomes so integrated into the family system of care that those offering assistance move into the private domain of family life. In such cases, friends can function very effectively by helping the caregiver without any expectation of being entertained or receiving the caring attention that a host or hostess normally gives guests. This total informality, which some informants described as having the quality of a pajama party—in that some people may be sleeping on the floor, and others in their nightclothes may be talking with the visitors—allows the caregiver to have the benefit of social contact with the outside without the strain of having to leave home or act as host or hostess.

> PAT KNOTT: When Lisa was in the hospital, one of our neighbors had a key, and we would come home and find our laundry freshly cleaned and folded. I mean she went up to our bedroom and took the dirty laundry, and so that when we came home we had fresh clothes to put on.

> ANNA KROLICK: These two friends of mine, Ed and Polly, would take turns coming almost every night about ten or eleven. They usually brought something sweet and would just come in and talk. It was right around the time when the late night shift had gone to bed and whoever was on the early shift was up alone. It helped to just sit around and eat cookies and talk about all the things that had happened that day and about our worries for Elizabeth. I really appreciated those visits.

Reciprocity

Most caregivers have less trouble accepting that others are making decisions for them or coming into their homes to do their laundry than accepting that all this is given without the expectation of a payback. Many caregivers struggled with this asymmetry. Some found more general ways to reciprocate, as these examples illustrate. One even founded her own hospice agency.

> BONNIE STEINER: There are a lot of people who, if it hadn't been for them, I don't know how I would have gotten through this, and I wanted to pay some of this back. I wanted to give to someone else because I don't know what I would have done if someone hadn't been willing to give to me. I became the coordinator of a support group for parents who had lost children and did this for several years.

> PAT KNOTT: I still actually, this many years later, have a hard time with that. There is a part of me that feels that I have to pay all these people back, and I know that the things that were given were not given with the intent that they ever be paid back. I still have a little trouble with that sometimes. I feel, "How in my life can I ever do what people did

for me, for us." And I can't. I mean I hope that those people never have a similar situation. It is hard to respond to but sometimes it is just really overwhelming to me, just real overwhelming to me what people did.

Those who provide social support do it for reasons that in most cases are largely symbolic. The support indicates the affection for and commitment to the dying person or caregiver. When it is aimed at the caregiver, it serves as a significant indicator that the person providing the assistance wishes to be part of the caregiver's life after the dying person is gone. People do not expect conventional reciprocity—a dinner for a dinner. Instead, supporters said things like, "I know you'd do this for me if I ever needed it," or "Help someone else who needs it."

Organizing a Support System

Families and those who helped them worked out systems of support which met the specific needs and capabilities of their unique situations. Some of the systems worked out by the informants in this book are described below. Some were formal and quite organized, like that of Pat Knott, and others were very informal.

STAN CLARK: One friend took Tuesdays as the day she could be a companion to Alice. We said to Alice's sister, "Could you do this?" and she wasn't sure if she could; but she came two mornings a week for several months. Then I had a friend who alternated with his wife coming mornings or afternoons. In fact one came in the morning and the other one in the afternoon. And there were two women friends of Alice's. People were either former students of hers or lifelong friends. So there were her two sisters, our daughters as they could fit it into their schedules every evening, and four or five other people who committed themselves to a morning or day per week. If for some reason they couldn't come they arranged to trade with someone else. They all knew the nurse and had talked with the doctor.

ANNA KROLICK: When Elizabeth was in the hospital near my sister, she and her husband took turns being at the hospital. When they needed a break, my brother flew in and took over. They were all clear that I should take my vacation because I would need it. When she was at my house, my sister or brother and their spouses took turns being here. Except for two or three days, one of them and often two were here. They took the 1 A.M. to 5 A.M. shift and let us get sleep. Then Elizabeth's best friend helped out by coming over occasionally during meals and sitting with her so we could eat together and have some time to discuss what was happening. Whoever wasn't here called every day, often several times, and was part of all the decisions.

FLORENCE MARTIN: My brother-in-law came two nights a week for six hours to let me get some sleep. The other nights, I hired the sixteen-year-old boy across the street to come over and help me get him ready for bed. I had two friends who would help me lift him. My daughter was here, but there were some things I did not feel my daughter should be doing, like helping him go to the bathroom. If something happened and I had to leave, a neighbor would come over and stay with him.

MARTHA QUINN: One of the absolute saving things about this whole experience has been the relationship of the three of us sisters which has [been] and continues to be terrific. When I think about trying to do this alone! We have sort of complemented each other well. I am the one with the youngest children and felt more immobilized and don't live very near, so I tended to do a lot of things that could be done by phone. Also, because I am in the mental health field, I have done a lot of contacts vis-à-vis my mother for hospitals and doctors and so forth. My sister who lived near and has one teenage son was closer physically to my parents, and more mobile, [and] did a lot of the literal legwork and helping with caretaking and going over to the house. And my sister from out-of-state just made lots of trips and did as much as she could down there but mostly came up for periods of time.

Table 1. Types of Support

Support for the Dying Person	Support for the Caregiver
By Family Members	**By Family Members**
Intimate care	Relief in caregiving
Nursing care	Participation in decision making
Reassurance	Financial support
Sitting with the person	Assumption of caregiver's other
Feeding	responsibilities
Administering medication	Attending to caregiver's health
	and well-being
	Communicating with others
	Assuming the care of other
	dependent family members

By Friends and Associates
Short, arranged visits
Cards
Video- and audiotapes
Photographs
Letters
Flowers
Scented or tactilely sensuous
    gifts

By Friends and Associates
Laundry
Meals
Transportation
Child care
Shopping
Cleaning
House maintenance
Car maintenance
Yard maintenance
Responsibilities at work
Visits/care of pets and plants

The Inclusion of Children

Children perceive and are aware of far more than they are able to talk or ask questions about. What they imagine is happening when a person is dying may be more frightening than the reality. For example, children may blame themselves for the illness and eventual death. It is far better to tell them as accurately as possible what is happening than to let them create explanations for themselves. Children are very sensitive to the behavior of the adults in their lives. They are aware of even subtle changes.

LAURA SWEET: When Tony was sick, he was so tired that he couldn't play with the children and they couldn't play with him because he was in so much pain. He was sensitive all over his body from the therapy, the nerve damage, and the incision in his chest. They could not give him a big hug. Kids aren't like that, they can't control themselves. I think they were standoffish because they didn't know what was going on and they were afraid.

Children don't need to be given all the details of what is happening. Once they have a basic understanding of the person's condition and know it is O.K. to discuss it, they will ask questions when they want to know something. Their questions can be a guide for the caregiver and dying person about how much information to provide. One thing they may not ask directly but will want to know is whether the caregiving parent is going to die, too. It is essential to reassure them that this won't happen. Very young children do not need a complicated explanation or to be told that the caregiver too will die some day. Their most immediate need is to be reassured, and it is not dishonest to tell them that the caregiver will not die and leave it at that.

Children should be included in activities with the dying person in as normal a manner as possible. This will help reassure them that their daily life has some continuity and stability.

> LUCILLE DeMOTT: We had a daily routine where the baby and Jim and I took care of medical visits while we tried to give Philip as normal a school routine as possible. We continued to do the things we used to do. We had a ritual of playing board games together. We continued to do that and had our music. It was a very highly interactive family time. I'd say that, except for the last month, life was as normal as it could have been under the circumstances. Life was routine; our family life was maintained.

The involvement with the dying person and his or her care can give children an immense sense of satisfaction. However, the child's ability to withdraw from the situation and not take any responsibility should be preserved.

> ANNA KROLICK: My daughter was just turning three when my mother died, but she still remembers the night when my mother was screaming with frightening hallucinations and woke her up. She came downstairs and gave her grandmother her teddy bear and my mother stopped screaming and became herself. She remembers she helped her grandmother when she needed it.

The extent to which children will want to be involved with the dying person will vary. Young children may be unaware of the strangeness of some of the physical changes, such as hair loss due to chemotherapy, which may upset slightly older children. Teenagers, who are just discovering their own body and sexuality, may be especially upset by the physical deterioration of the dying person. When given the choice, most children will make clear when they want to be with the patient and when they don't. Their wishes should be respected.

> LUCILLE DeMOTT: We asked Philip how he wanted to do many things. There came a point when he wanted to leave the house. He couldn't

stand to watch his father die. We found someone to take him, one of his friends' family. He lived there for a week. Then the mom called and said he wanted to come home. I talked to him, and I said, "That's fine." He came home, and as it was obvious that this week was the death week and—he did not want to leave, he just didn't. He just spent a lot of time hugging his dad.

HELENA WOLF: Herbert went into the hospital sort of precipitously. When the kids came home from school, he had gone into the hospital. We talked about whether they should go to the hospital that night to see him. They both said they would go if we wanted them to. Gregg said, "I'll go if you want me to." I said, "No." I had no need for them to go. I could understand, and they didn't want to go, and I think it was the right decision. I'm not a believer in this saying goodbye.

The presence of children can be an immense source of comfort for the dying. Children can give unconditional love and attachment. They also represent the future.

LUCILLE DEMOTT: When Jim was sick in the hospital, I told Philip I didn't know what would happen. Sometimes he would decide to spend the night in the hospital with me. He would climb into bed with Jim and urge him to live, and he was there when Jim first regained consciousness. There was a lot of just lying in bed and hugging and kissing. We were a three-person support team. The kids, both kids were there all day so that Jim could see them and they could see him.

ANNA KROLICK: Almost the only time my mother could pull herself together and be herself was when my daughter was around. They were very attached to each other, and she would play on Mother's bed and Mother would talk to her the way she always had. At night when she was so agitated, Mother would call for her and whenever she saw her she managed to smile. It was quite remarkable because she really seemed demented a lot of the time, and yet she could be completely appropriate when my daughter was there.

In some cases, the presence of children can create a painful reminder of how much the dying person is leaving behind.

HELENA WOLF: The kids were the most difficult problem, very difficult. They had a very close relationship with him and they would go to his room every day. It became increasingly clear that he didn't want to see them. He made it be known very clearly that he just couldn't see them; it was just painful, it was the one recognition of his mortality. Somehow with me it wasn't the same. He just couldn't cope with knowing that he wouldn't see them grow up. It was just too painful.

Problems in the Support System

Tending the terminally ill is an extremely intense experience; it can be expected to raise strong emotions, emotions concerning people's relationship to the dying person, to the main caregiver, and to one another, as well as their own feelings of adequacy, power, courage, and loss. Antagonisms, fears, weaknesses, and conflicts with long histories emerge along with the strength and courage it takes to care for a dying person. Some problems are resolved and bring people closer together. Others are exacerbated, creating a permanent barrier.

It is impossible to establish a set of guidelines for dealing with the disputes and emotional problems arising from such a stressful undertaking and intense time in people's lives. Far too many issues hidden and overt will be involved. The problems the informants faced illustrate some of the reasons they were so upsetting. There are roughly three kinds of problems: 1) people who take more than they give; 2) expected social support that fails to materialize; and 3) support that unintentionally undermines the caregiver.

When Support Doesn't Work

Visits by people whom the caregiver and other close family members must host are usually prearranged and limited in duration. In this way the caregiver tries to control the stress of having to host people. Problems can arise when people who are admitted into the informal sphere of family life of those doing the caregiving expect to be treated as guests. Instead of offering relief, they put additional pressures on the caregivers. These tend to be people who are permitted to visit in a more flexible fashion, such as relatives or old family friends, and it is assumed that they are committed to the caregiver— and thus mindful of his or her well-being—as well as to the dying person. When they are not committed to the caregiver or when their own needs are so great they demand attention from the caregiver, their support drains rather than replenishes.

This can also be a problem when caring for an acutely ill person in the hospital. Except in the intensive care unit, there are far fewer constraints on visitors in the hospital than in the home. People, in fact, feel an obligation to visit. But for the caregiver and the patient, if alert, these visits can be a strain. It is wise to call the caregiver first to confirm that a visit would be appreciated and determine how long it should be. If a potential supporter is discouraged from visiting, this should be interpreted not as a rejection but rather as an indication of the stress the caregiver and patient are under. One can find other ways of showing that one cares, such as dropping a meal or bag of groceries off at the caregiver's home.

People mean well when they try to comfort and support the caregiver, but those actions can sometimes go wrong.

BONNIE STEINER: One woman came up to me at the funeral and said, "Well, I think you and Jack ought to go right home and make another baby." I wanted to smack her across the face. My best friend heard the comment and it was all I could do to keep her away from the woman. People make such inane comments like "You can always have more children" or "I think you ought to have another baby right away."

Unless the person offering support has actually been through a very similar experience, it is better not to say, "I know how you feel." The intensity of home death is difficult to imagine for those who have not been part of it. A more helpful approach is to provide opportunities for the caregiver to talk and to indicate that even though the supporter can't understand, he or she feels deeply for the caregiver.

PAT KNOTT: I don't know if I will save these forever, but we never didn't get a card in the mail, and many days we got many cards. A lot came from a circle of friends and from family members. It is helpful to know that people are thinking about you even if they can't be there—letting you know in some way that they are with you. It was very helpful when people said things like, "I can't really understand what you are going through but I want you to know I am thinking of you all the time."

BONNIE STEINER: I would have liked to have more people say, "I am here if you want to talk, I am here." Then if we were together, ask me, "Do you want to talk about it?" and then let me sit there and cry, and cry with me.

Lack of Social Support

All the informants in this study decided to care for the dying person at home with the expectation that friends and family would in some way help. Everyone received assistance to some extent, but there were many cases where it was not forthcoming—at least not to the degree needed by the caregiver. Permanent strains in friendships and rifts in families resulted.

There are many reasons why someone the caregiver expects to provide support may be unable or unwilling to do so. Sometimes people may be very afraid of the disease, especially if they themselves have had it or had an experience with it.

> MARY ROEHM: One friend was very good with Carl because he would sit with him and visit and get him to talk because he had more stories that he could tell. No other friends helped out regularly. We had some really good friends but they rarely came. One good friend just couldn't face it; his father had had Alzheimer's and he couldn't face it. It bothered Carl a lot that this man didn't come, but he just couldn't face it.

When the dying person suffers from AIDS, the fear of the disease combined with the disapproval people may feel for the practices that can lead to it can rob the caregiver of potential support in caring for the dying person. The stigma works two ways: it may prevent the dying person or caregiver from disclosing the true nature and seriousness of the illness, and it may drive away potential helpers. Lucinda Klein faced this double problem:

> My parents are in Minnesota and my brother is in Connecticut. He was the one member of my family who knew Joyce, but she didn't want him to know she had AIDS. My mother knew Joyce was very, very sick. My mother didn't want my father to know we were lovers, so he never knew. My parents did know that my friend Joyce had been very sick and was now living with me. My father was warmer, but he knew less about our relationship. He said he was very proud of me. The whole thing with friends was complicated by the fact that Joyce and I were lesbians, and lesbians don't usually get AIDS unless from drug use. She didn't want people to know that about her, that she had been a drug addict, which I understand entirely. But they all know now. She

couldn't tell them one thing without the other. I told a few of our friends that she had AIDS, because I had to tell someone. Those friends came real often, once a week, and that was real nice.

In some situations, the friends of the dying person may feel they can't intrude on the home of the caregiver when they are not close friends with that person. This may occur when an adult child is caring for a parent. It sometimes happens when the wife is dying and the husband's friends feel they can't intrude in another woman's home. One woman informant who had helped care for a dying person said:

When Mary's husband was sick, I thought nothing of going over to help. But when Peter's wife got sick, even though he and I are good friends, I didn't think of going over there. And now, thinking about it, I know I would have felt uncomfortable because it was her house and I would have been intruding.

In some cases it is the dying person who prevents the caregiver from receiving support. When the dying person has not yet come to terms with death, he or she may not be able to confront the affirmation of what is happening by discussing it with others or even having others visit when that signifies recognition of the terminal illness. For these patients, controlling the information of their terminal illness may be one of the few areas over which they can still exercise control. These people may insist that no one be told, which is what Herbert Wolf demanded, at least initially.

HELENA WOLF: He didn't want people to know, which was very strange and put me in a very bizarre kind of situation. People obviously began to know, and for a while, when he was here and still sitting up, people wanted to come and see him. He wouldn't let people come and I sort of got to be the go-between. I think you just have to respect people's wishes. Toward the end this got to be excruciatingly difficult.

He would sort of send me out and say, "O.K., you can go and tell X." Then I would get to go and tell whomever he had identified. "O.K., you go and tell so and so that I won't be coming around." So we would have these events where I would go and tell someone and invariably they would write him a note, and I would have to read him the note. Excruciating, as you can imagine, for everyone involved.

That is something you have to weigh; that is one of the big issues to weigh: your needs as a caregiver as opposed to the needs of the patient.

The person who is actually dying will want interaction in some cases and in other cases the support will have to go primarily to the family, to the people helping out.

When family members do not supply the expected support, the potential problems are much more serious. Longstanding conflicts and tensions can impede the family from functioning effectively to care for the dying person. This does not mean that every family member needs to perform the same amount or kind of work. Most families described here were able to divide tasks according to the abilities of the various individuals. Problems occurred when people who were perceived as perfectly able to help for some reason did not, or did so in a very inadequate fashion.

BONNIE STEINER: My sister called four or five times. She wouldn't even come up, even when I said, "Betty, I need you to come. I need you to come here." "Well, I have a cold." "Well, we can meet somewhere else; Jack can stay with David." Well, she wouldn't do it. Well, I don't think I spoke to her for a year. Five years later I am still very resentful of her, still having trouble dealing with the anger.

Caregivers reported being shocked by the lack of assistance, especially when family relationships previously had been cordial. One possible explanation that seems to hold for the cases reported here is that the people who fail to offer social support do not see themselves in an enduring relationship to the caregiver. Most of the caregivers who were disappointed were remarried wives and one fiancée who failed to receive adequate care from their partner's family.

LAURA SWEET: His family needed to be more involved. His mother worked for the state. When he died she had 240 sick days left. She had all that time accumulated which she could have taken to be with him, but she didn't. I had five sick days, which I blew right away. His sister disappointed me to the point that I finally said something to his mother because she never came down at all. She never called. She never wrote him a card.

LUCILLE DeMOTT: I have had no contact with those children since the funeral. I haven't desired contact. They chose not to come to the funeral even though they knew he had planned the ceremony. They did that to hurt me. Certainly they weren't hurting him. They made a very clear statement that they didn't want to be involved with me and my children.

FLORENCE MARTIN: His children came to help sometimes, except for one who didn't live around here and the one who couldn't handle it, so we saw very little of her. He had three brothers and three sisters and a mother [aged] eighty who doesn't drive, so she wasn't any help. His one sister and two brothers live within fifty miles. One was having a baby so she couldn't come. The other siblings did not come. He had a sister in Florida who made six trips to see him. I would have liked more help from anybody. The children were impossible—but at least his family—but they did not help. It was like he had the plague. Here one sister will come thousands of miles to see him, but a brother who only lives thirty miles away won't. It was not even to help me so much as that he needed them.

Because of a long period in which deaths occurred mainly in hospitals, our society has few conventions for dealing with the dying at home. There are numerous reasons why people fail to provide expected support. Many are not able to confront death so intimately. Some are simply afraid of death and reject any contact with it. Others are afraid of the particular disease. Still others feel they can't intrude on the home. Lack of support for the dying person should not be seen as an indication of the quality of the person's relationship to that person. Assistance for the caregiver is somewhat different in that actions taken or not taken will be remembered and become a part of the relationship in the future.

People's actions and attitudes surrounding the care of the terminally ill are not isolated but instead reflect their past relationships and feelings, and the actions of the patient as well as the caregiver. It is not possible to separate the dying person or caregiver from his or her history. Many of the problems in lack of support can be traced to this history. Social workers attached to hospices or home care agencies clearly can be especially helpful in identifying and possibly resolving these longstanding problems. A neutral party can help negotiate areas of conflict and arrive at workable solutions for providing care and supporting the caregiver. (See chapter 3 for a more detailed discussion of these problems.)

Social support is one of the most important factors in determining how successful an experience home death will be for both the dying person and the caregiver and how strained the latter will be after the person dies. At this emotionally highly charged time, large and small gestures take on significance for the caregiver beyond the gift or assistance provided. Social support can affirm for both that they are important members of the social community. For the caregiver in this time of need, loss, and grief the bond created by social support remains strong.

CHAPTER FIVE

The Well-being of the Caregiver

People would say, "You have to get some sleep." And I would say, "I can sleep after he dies. I just can't think about myself. If he is more comfortable when I am there, I will be there. I can't be away; I can't sleep." I was really driven.

—BONNIE STEINER

The caregiver is the key element in making home death possible. On the caregiver's shoulders rests the responsibility for the dying person's well-being. Formal support provided by organizations such as hospice and informal support from friends, colleagues, and neighbors can be an invaluable additional resource; but it is the caregiver who must assume primary responsibility for making the system work. Like a distance runner, caregivers must preserve their strength and pace themselves. This chapter examines the nature of the strains—physical and emotional—that caregivers experience and details the various ways those in this study dealt with them. It goes on to describe why caregivers feel they were capable of assuming this responsibility and concludes with their evaluation of the experience.

Day to Day

Those caregivers who had never tended a dying person were struck by how different the experience was from what they had envisioned. It was both more strenuous and less intimidating. The sheer physical effort was surprising—sometimes overwhelming. At the same time, in part precisely because the physical demands were so great, the clear awareness of what was actually happening—that one was caring for someone who was about to die and would in all probability die in one's presence—was often absent.

The image of impending death as dominating all aspects of life failed to emerge in a context where the caregiver was immersed in and responsible for the mechanics of caring for an acutely ill person at home. The caregiver's desire to allow the person to live out the remainder of life as a person, not as a "patient," was realized through the actual performance of caregiving. The day-to-day demands took on a structure and rhythm of their own. They came to define the lives of both the caregiver and the dying person and as such kept the immediate awareness of death at a distance.

Ironically, the caregivers' lives became almost simple. They described a process in which their priorities were clearly ordered, with caring for the dying person taking first place, followed by care for other dependent people. What little energy was left went to meeting other responsibilities. This ordering of priorities removed the need most people had to choose constantly among the various things that needed to be done. Some spoke of a kind of peaceful simplicity and calm that descended on their lives as they abandoned other roles and responsibilities and focused exclusively on caregiving. This calm was of course juxtaposed with the extreme stress they were under, the sacrifices that terminal care demanded of them, and the overwhelming nature of the fatigue and strain.

The descriptions of day-to-day life which follow illustrate the engrossing character of this care and the way it helped protect those giving it from confronting the stark nature of their undertaking: to help the person they loved to die.

> HELENA WOLF: Your emotional unconscious protects you from what is happening. You focus on what needs to be done today: "What are we going to eat? Wouldn't it be fun to have this? Later on so and so is going to come over." You shut out for yourself that this is happening in a continuum because you can't perceive that it is happening over the long term. In that sense it is like taking care of a small baby because you fall into an incredibly simplistic routine that involves making meals, picking up from them, making coffee, and "Which cracker will we eat now? Are we going to take a bath?" and "Let's comb your hair." And it becomes very complete. It takes all day to do those things. I certainly had no sense of this terrible void—here are going to be all these hours. You are both protected and you become very isolated.

Maintaining a daily routine helped people cope with the strain of acute caregiving. It may seem, and it may be the case, that one's world is being torn asunder, yet when there is a certain predictabil-

ity to each day's events, when everyone sits down to dinner together, when birthdays are still celebrated, albeit in the dying
person's room, life retains some familiar and reassuring qualities. It
is just this sense of familiarity and control over one's life and environment which death radically challenges, which is in part why it is
so frightening for most people. Maintaining a routine, observing
family rituals, help caregivers cope with pressures by making some
of the unknown familiar.

> HELENA WOLF: I think you enter a very protective mode where you
> discard the large picture because the large picture is overwhelming, and
> you become very preoccupied with "How is he feeling right now: are
> we going to get through this day?" and not "Oh my God, my father is
> dying."

Abstractly considered, the idea of caring for someone dying at
home focuses primarily on the idea of death. The abstraction of
death and the reality of impending loss color attempts by caregivers
to imagine what taking care of the dying person will be like. In
practice, caring for the dying is very much about life and helping the
dying person to live out what is left of life. In most cases, the fact of
death remained in the background, crowded out by the intense demands of caregiving.

The caregiver's commitment to helping the person live out the
rest of his or her life with the best quality of life possible meant that
the caregiver was often faced with innumerable decisions that had
to be made in the process of maintaining the patient's quality of life:
How should the medications be adjusted? What does this symptom
mean? Is death near, or is this a problem that can be reversed?
Should so-and-so be allowed to visit? What effect would a phone
call from so-and-so have? Will the patient be able to swallow this
kind of drink? How can I get him or her to eat something? To take
medicine? To sleep? Although making the decisions was a serious
and sometimes frightening responsibility, the constant barrage of
them provided an engrossing preoccupation that served to camou-
flage the fact of impending death.

> STAN CLARK: I can see that I existed by being able to solve those kinds of
> problems and I was able to avoid worrying about Alice's dying and my
> life after losing her.

Thus despite the fact that caregivers were engaged in tending the dying, death was somewhat unreal. Indeed, many had thought they were prepared for the death and nonetheless were surprised when it eventually came.

> HELENA WOLF: As realistic as it is to everyone around you—like if your next door neighbor tells you that their mother is dying, you say, "Oh I guess they are going to die"—but when it is happening to you it has no time frame; it is just happening. I always used to say that I felt that I was on an express train going someplace but I didn't know where I was going or when I was going to get there and it doesn't stop. It becomes all and totally engrossing.

> HELEN WRIGHT: I really—you really don't have time to think about the death. There was just so much to be done, each moment to do the best you could do. I knew it was happening or I wouldn't have told the children to come.

Terminal care is almost always a tremendous physical and emotional strain for the caregiver. This is so despite the often considerable help of outsiders, both professionals and friends. It is the caregiver who has the ultimate responsibility for care, and it is in the caregiver's family that the death is occurring.

The well-worn platitude "Take care of yourself" seems both too obvious and too trivial to discuss in this context. Yet it becomes a crucial issue for most caregivers. In the eyes of most of the informants, the needs of the dying person took absolute priority. As the caregiving progressed, however, many began to wear down, become exhausted, and burned out. Some faced the possibility that they would have to stop caring for the patient at home. As caregivers began to confront and experience their physical and emotional limits, they had to accept the need to care for themselves so they could continue to care for the dying person. Despite the compelling needs of the dying, caregivers, too, needed rest and comfort.

The Physical Drain

Informants initially expected that grief and the sense of impending loss would be the most difficult problem they would confront. Few caregivers expected the strenuous physical demands this task would place on them. The sheer physical effort was a major drain. Most people suffered from exhaustion; two developed back problems, and one had to be hospitalized.

The bedridden had to be turned every three hours to prevent bedsores, lifted and arranged in bed, transferred to the wheelchair, and helped with elimination and bathing. In many cases the caregiver provided physical therapy treatments and gave medications. Sometimes they performed technical procedures such as suctioning. And there was the ever present exhaustion, some of it nervous exhaustion, but much of it due simply to the lack of sleep.

HELENA WOLF: I basically stopped eating and stopped sleeping. Only later did I realize I was doing this. I would sit down at dinner and say, "Oh, there were some other meals today; what happened to those? Oh, it's dinner time; I should eat this."

LAURA SWEET: I guess I probably could not have gone on much longer. There was a point when, regardless of whether there was a nurse there or not, I was being woken up, so I wasn't getting more than two or three hours of sleep at a time. After a week or two, I started losing it. Sometimes, at night, Tony and I would just talk. Whenever he wanted to talk I would talk. There was a point [when] I was ready to collapse, and I called the agency head to send someone and went off and slept for a couple of days straight.

LUCILLE DeMOTT: I got very ill while caring for Jim and ended up with physical problems from a combination of stress, high blood pressure, and physical work. I had no idea I was hurting my body. People came in to treat the patient, to tell me about caring for his body but didn't caution me or train me to care for myself. It is amazing about how unperceptive one is at that time. So many health professionals are visiting the patient with you in the same room and no one notices you. I didn't even notice what was happening to me.

JOE STEAD: I would sleep a little, but if she turned over in bed, I was wide awake. It was real rough and I was going downhill. I got to where I felt I hadn't slept in forty-eight hours. When you get that bad, you shouldn't be there anyways. My daughter came over and stayed one night and that took the pressure off.

Despite the extreme stress the caregivers were under and the chronic sleep deprivation, they seemed immune to the more common ailments such as colds or flu. Many informants feared that they would get sick, or their health would give out and make it impossible for them to care for the dying person. With few exceptions, this did not happen. In fact, caregivers reported surprisingly good health, and two of them, one of whom suffered from chronic migraine headaches and the other from a back ailment, were not troubled at all by these problems during the period of caregiving.

To be able to continue providing effective care, making the decisions, and meeting the other demands placed on them, caregivers need to maintain some degree of normalcy. The longer the crisis lasts, the more normal life must become. People need normalcy in order to sustain this effort. Sleep is as fundamental as food for the caregiver. If, as frequently happens, the dying person does not sleep or sleeps irregularly or fitfully, there must be some relief so the caregiver can sleep. Some reported that they were able to sleep despite the disturbance created by the dying person, whereas others shut the bedroom door or slept in another part of the house when someone could be there to watch the patient. In a crisis, the best sleep can be obtained by actually leaving the house and going to a friend's or to a motel to sleep through one or two nights. If the caregiver must remain at home, it may be helpful to turn on the air conditioner or another noise-making device to cover the noise of the person who is dying. Sleep deprivation causes serious mental and physical impairment. It has even been used as a form of torture. The task facing the caregiver is extremely difficult and need not be made more so by prolonged shortage of sleep.

A great many people are not physically fit. Furthermore, *anyone* can easily sustain injury during caregiving without proper training. Even someone who is in good shape can be injured by performing one of these tasks improperly. If one has any particular physical limitations, these need to be taken into consideration in arranging supplemental help. Florence Martin, for instance, had had a mastectomy and knew her left arm was weak. To compensate, she arranged for a neighborhood boy to help her get her husband into bed every night.

The patient will continue to get worse, need more care, become more dependent. If the caregiver plans to care for the dying person until the end, he or she needs to take care too. Nutritious food, adequate sleep, exercise, and some form of break are essential. This is not the time for diets. Some caregivers modified their exercise so they could do something compatible with caregiving at home, such as yoga. Caregivers need to treat themselves with the realization that they are undergoing the most significant endurance event of their lives.

The Emotional Strain

Caring for the dying is an emotionally charged activity in which a whole range of feelings are experienced and expressed intensely. Caregivers describe a deep emotional satisfaction in having done something very significant for the dying person, often making possible the fulfillment of his or her specific wish to die at home. New depths of love, understanding, and appreciation may be reached between the two. At the same time, the caregiver may experience feelings of anger, guilt, fear, loneliness, depression, and a profound sense that one's life has been dislocated.

Grief

Many caregivers are so overwhelmed with fatigue that they experience a kind of emotional numbness. Although they are intimately involved in the dying process, they do not actively grieve until after the person dies. The anticipatory grieving that can happen in hospitals, where the family does not have the responsibility of day-to-day care and can withdraw from the patient, was rarely experienced by the caregivers in this study. In one case, however, the wife became so preoccupied with her grieving that she was no longer able to care for her husband. Instead she spent the day on the telephone—sometimes ten hours a day—talking with friends about coping with her husband's death while her sister-in-law and son cared for the dying man.

Caregivers saw the decision to give terminal care at home as an affirmation of life. It is, therefore, not surprising that they did not focus on grief. In the midst of death their focus was on life. Active caregiving kept them emotionally and psychologically involved with the person until death occurred. Their lack of anticipatory grieving is similar to that reported in *The Hospice Experiment* (Mor et al. 1988) of caregivers who nursed the dying at home. With the exception of Florence Martin, the caregivers interviewed for this book were surprised when death actually came. They had not permitted themselves the emotional distance that comes with grief.

HELEN WRIGHT: I think there is some denial in there. You can't really face what it means to die. After he died, I felt, "I wish I had been a little more aware that he was going to die so soon." Because it had gone on so long, for so many months that it seemed that it might go on forever. I was sure the woman who came to stay the night would be needed. I buzzed around getting things ready for her. I had expected him to live through the night, so it was a surprise that he *didn't* live through the night.

Intermittent caregivers, those who came in to relieve the main one, had more difficulty remaining engaged with the dying person. In the time when they were not actively participating, they began to grieve, only to be brought back into contact when they resumed their caregiving. They were unable to sustain the almost protective denial of the main caregiver. This was a particularly difficult problem for Anna Krolick's brother, who, on his last visit to his mother, was unable to spend much time in her room. Instead he took over managing the house, arranging schedules of other supporters, and attended to legal and financial matters.

Lack of Control

Although caregivers may not confront death directly, they must constantly struggle with the implications of death: namely, that human beings in many ways have very little control over their lives. This is one of the most fear-inspiring aspects of death. Much of life is possible only because we impose on it some order and predictability—which are invented by human beings. Time is an example of a convention created by humans to establish order. Natural forces also continually intervene and disrupt that order. When these disruptions occur, they are upsetting in part because they demonstrate our lack of control over life. Often they can be corrected, lives put back together, buildings rebuilt. Death, however, is final and cannot be reversed. It is perhaps the most profound indication that life is not under our control.

Caregivers confront the loss of control on two levels. There is the abstract yet intimate knowledge that death is about to occur and that nothing can be done to stop it. There is also the day-to-day struggle to try to impose some order on life. Despite the absolutely compelling nature of this kind of caregiving and the protective immersion this intensity offers, many caregivers are faced with the need—often coming from the outside—to attempt to impose some order on life. It is especially difficult for those who also have responsibilities such as a job or children or both.

Although physicians or nurses cannot say for sure when someone will die, many caregivers feel a need to anticipate the person's death, to be able to ration their energies and the support they are receiving from others. Caregivers must balance the need to impose some order on the situation with the knowledge that it is inherently unstable and unpredictable. This is, of course, extremely difficult, because planning implies that one has accepted and anticipated the death; it thus impels caregivers to shed their self-protective immersion. Caregivers were concerned that the very act of planning might diminish their commitment to the dying person. Yet plans have to be made, especially in prolonged caregiving. Many informants were torn by this dilemma.

> HELENA WOLF: My overwhelming memory was this concept of time. I wondered how long it would be; how long the different phases would last. Would he be weak and bedridden? Would he become incontinent? Would he need to be fed? And some sense of how long it was going to be. One of the most frightening things is this sense of open-endedness. Nobody tells you. It's not that they don't tell you; they just don't know. So you are looking forward into this void. That was very hard.
>
> If it had turned out to be longer, I would have started thinking in some kind of increments. "Let's have a plan for the next two weeks," and "This is who will help out," and then reevaluate at the end of two weeks rather than try to deal with it on a day-to-day basis. I would try to see things in some sort of units and have some evaluation because, if you perceive it as a void, it is so overwhelming that you can't continue as the person gets sicker and sicker but doesn't die. You have to have some way of measuring your own strength, your own resources.

Hospice workers can help caregivers think through the likely course of events and help them prepare themselves for the demands of caregiving. Although they can't predict exactly what will happen, hospice workers can describe and identify the different stages. If the caregiver can develop a daily routine, the sense of crisis will be alleviated and a sense of control will be introduced. Planning helps the caregiver cope with the uncertainty; nevertheless, the caregiver must remain flexible in order to be able to adapt to unexpected developments.

The dying person may also experience an intense sense of loss of control. On the other hand, some who accept their death are able to exercise control over their lives by organizing their death, choosing the place of death, putting their affairs in order, even orchestrating their own funeral. Those who do not come to terms with death, however, may become extremely angry over the loss of control in their lives.

Anger

The anger of the dying person is one of the most difficult emotions caregivers have to confront. For the most part, caregivers interviewed for this book did not feel free to respond to the anger in the way they normally would. They saw the dying person as extremely vulnerable and dependent, which of course is an accurate perception. They felt so constrained by the fact that they were going to live and the dying person was not that this overwhelming discrepancy in their lives made it almost impossible to respond to the anger unless they were extremely provoked. As Lucinda Klein said, "I just stood there and took it." This inability to respond, this feeling that one had to "swallow" one's feelings, created serious strain in some caregivers which was exacerbated by the anxiety that the dying person did not appreciate what the caregiver was doing.

Dying people may vent their anger by trying to control the caregiver, placing absurd and unrelenting demands on the caregiver and retaliating furiously when these demands are not met.

> FLORENCE MARTIN: He was very nasty, very nasty. The lady who came in said he was like Dr. Jekyll or Mr. Hyde whenever I or my daughter came in the room. He was angry because he was dying and we were living. We were to sit there and not leave the room and watch him die; that is what he wanted. No matter what you did, it was wrong. It was his way of control. He believed he had complete control over his life and anything that happened to him was his fault. All of a sudden he got this disease, which was not his fault, which he could not control, and it just completely destroyed his belief in everything. Consequently, he tried to control everybody else. I probably let him do that also because I felt so bad because he was dying and felt that was one of the things he could still do was control me.

Sometimes this anger is an extension of a long-term pattern of hostility in the relationship. Sometimes it is a completely new development, and then it may be even more deeply disturbing to the caregivers, who believed they knew the dying person and understood who he or she was.

Controlling the caregiver is an immediate, almost tangible expression of the dying person's continued ability to have an effect on life; to have some things, even very small things, go according to his or her desires. Because caregivers are acutely aware of the vulnerability of the dying, they find it extremely difficult to respond assertively to the anger. They see no point in "drawing the line" because they have no intention of abandoning the person.

> LUCINDA KLEIN: She would be just so angry. I would yell back. We always had arguments. I just don't know what you do with that anger. The leader of the support group said to me, "So what is your bottom line?" I said, "What do you mean, bottom line? She is my lover; she has AIDS; do you think I am going to throw her out?" My bottom line was that I was going to keep taking care of her.

As long as the caregiver judged the dying person to be rational, the caregiver continuously struggled with a mixture of guilt, hurt, and resentment, as well as a protective sympathy. When the patient was cognitively impaired, the anger was less threatening but still painful. In some cases, cognitive impairment resulting from the disease can accompany the dying process and can cause hallucinations; it can also break down inhibitions about expressing feelings, including anger. Anna Krolick was never sure whether her mother's anger was from the **brain metastases,** from her refusal to accept death, or from a decision she made to tell people exactly what she thought. For whatever reason, Elizabeth was angry much of the time.

> ANNA KROLICK: She would say some pretty horrible things. Towards the end she wouldn't even let my husband come near her; she was so mad at him. Some of what she said had some truth in it, so it was hard to know what to do with it. Sometimes she apologized and said the codeine made her say things, but it could be pretty awful.

Although the anger is directed *at* the caregiver, it often isn't really *about* the caregiver. It represents rage at having to die and sometimes anger that family members will survive. This is especially a problem between spouses and other life partners. In some cases the anger reflects the person's utter dependence on the caregiver and the fear of being abandoned.

LUCINDA KLEIN: You can reassure a person only so much. You don't know if they really believe you. She was abandoned as a kid. If I was that sick, I would be afraid that they would abandon me at some point. Because why should they stick around? It seems very unequal and demanding on one side.

The manipulative behavior that may accompany the anger is the dying person's way of reclaiming control over a life rapidly careening out of control. Trying to give the dying person control over caregiving decisions helps relieve some anger. But when this compromises the caregiver's ability to go on, such as when Florence Martin's husband refused to let her leave the house, the caregiver needs to take some protective action.

The clergy or the hospice workers who specialize in helping the dying come to terms with death can help relieve this anger. If the caregiver suspects that the anger may derive from medication or the underlying disease process (hospice personnel should be able to help diagnose this), it helps to reassure the patient that what is happening is caused by the disease and that the caregivers understand this.

Fear of Death

Although most caregivers denied death to the extent that they did not actively begin grieving until the person actually died, they did try to anticipate what the death would be like. They asked doctors and nurses what to expect so they could prepare themselves. Hospices in particular were able to supply information about the signs and symptoms of approaching death, and about death itself. For people who had never experienced a death before, this information was sometimes insufficient to calm their fears, and they remained anxious and fearful.

HELENA WOLF: It was a constant dread—going away and having to come back, even if I came back right away, that I might go over there and find him dead. That became more and more of a barrier. It doesn't mean I didn't go; but you thought about it all the time. There was always the fear he would go to sleep and die. Once he went to the hospital, it became even more overwhelming. It's just there on your mind.

LAURA SWEET: I had read about **Cheyne-Stokes** breathing, but it didn't say when he would do it. So the last two months, I couldn't sleep because I was listening for this breathing. I really thought (we didn't have anyone at night) that he was going to die and I would be the only person there in the apartment. I was terrified. I would not go from room to room without the light on. I was afraid of the dark. It was spooky. I was afraid of death. I was afraid of him dying, I was afraid of waking up next to a dead stiff body. I was terrified. Luckily, that is not the way it happened.

Fear of the actual death is one of the main reasons people rehospitalize the patient at the point of death or refuse to care for the dying at home. In large part this is because Americans are unfamiliar with death. Because hospitals have become the primary site of death over the last fifty years, people have little intimate experience with it. Thus, death is mysterious and frightening.

Although no one can say exactly when a person will die, there are clear signs that death is near. Some, such as changes in breathing patterns (see chapter 6), may occur and then stop. In such cases many people prepare themselves for the death only to have the patient pull through; then the caregiver must readjust to the continued need for caregiving. But when several signs occur together, the likelihood that death is imminent is greatly increased. In most cases trained hospice personnel can predict death within a range of several days, which allows caregivers to prepare themselves for the likelihood that death will come soon. The possibility that death will take everyone by surprise is not high when a person is dying at home. Caregivers need not frighten themselves with the image of coming upon death suddenly. Although it is always a possibility, the sudden, unpredicted death of a patient cared for by a hospice is unlikely.

Hospice personnel can do much to alleviate the fear of sudden, unanticipated death. They provide written information about the signs and symptoms of approaching death and talk with the caregivers about what to expect. Perhaps most importantly, they make a very serious effort to be in the home when the person dies to help the caregiver, other family members, and the dying person through this process. Their presence can have a significant reassuring effect on those present. They can explain what the different stages of dying are. They also counsel the family on how to respond to the dying person. Typically they suggest that the family gather around, hold the dying person's hand, talk about their love for him or her. The hospice worker also confirms that death has occurred—something that may be difficult to determine for lay people if, for example, the patient was comatose.

People die in many different ways (see chapter 6), none of them beyond the bounds of natural experience—none is supernatural. The room is not filled with the ghostly presence of the dead person; no cold wind blows. Death often comes, during sleep or a coma, when a person stops breathing. Some deaths are more agonized, for example, when the heart stops. But death is not unworldly.

Responsibilities to Others

With so much attention focused on the dying person and all the emotional and psychological imperatives created by imminent death, it is difficult for the caregiver to fulfill responsibilities to others. The others may be a spouse, dependent children, or a dependent parent or older relative. All of these people have a legitimate need for the caregiver's attention. Their needs, however, can constitute additional, sometimes intolerable, burdens for the caregiver.

Children

Children are very difficult for a parent to ignore. Depending on their ages and personalities, their needs may be either constant or intermittent. Almost all will need at least emotional contact with the caregiving parent. Even if one can provide little else, one should make every attempt to sustain emotional contact with the child. Children will be frightened by the parent's preoccupation and will need to be reassured that the caregiving parent is not dying and still thinks about and cares about them even if he or she cannot be there for them at this time.

Children will benefit to the extent that the normal daily household routine can be maintained. If familiar people—friends, neighbors, other relatives—can help entertain and care for them, the children may be somewhat reassured. Familiar patterns provide very concrete reassurances to children that their world is still intact. They will also need to ask questions about what is happening. If the caregiving parent is unable to answer them, the social worker at the hospice can help. An outside therapist can also be an invaluable resource. Outside help, in the form of either advice for the parent or support for the child, is especially important if the dying person is the other parent. (See appendix B for resources to use in dealing with this problem.)

Children can also be an enormous source of respite during this time. Their very concrete involvement in everyday activities is a refreshing break from the existential issues of death. To attend to their needs in even a minimal way, the caregiver must make sufficient time to focus on them and put the dying person's needs at a distance temporarily.

Even very young children have a surprising ability to maintain their equilibrium, to keep themselves "together," in a crisis. The effect it is having on them may not be noticeable until after the immediate crisis has passed and they feel secure enough to express their feelings. Getting children, even young children, to ask questions about what is happening, answering their questions, and providing explanations appropriate to their age can help them cope with the crisis and reduce problems they may encounter later.

Parents

Middle-aged Americans are increasingly taking on the responsibility of caring for their aging parents, who to a greater or lesser extent need help in daily living. During the time a person is caring for someone who is dying, relatives may be able to assume the caregiver's duties in caring for the parent. If this is not possible, local social service agencies such as Adult Protective Services may be able to suggest sources of substitute help. These substitute caregivers will probably have to be paid, although churches and volunteer organizations are sometimes able to provide short-term help at no charge or for a nominal donation.

Caregivers face a more serious problem when the dying person is also the main support of the elderly parent or relative. When this happens, the caregiver must either assume the care of two people—which is beyond the abilities of most people—or consider significant outside help. This is a situation where nursing home placement might be necessary. Martha Quinn encountered a particularly difficult problem when her father developed terminal cancer and she and her sisters discovered the extent of their mother's mental illness.

MARTHA QUINN: My mother has an extensive psychiatric history and for the last ten years has been in pretty rough shape. After my father retired, taking care of her became his full-time job. He did the cooking, laundry, shopping, and driving. After he had gotten sick, my sisters and I were incredulous of what he had done to maintain her at home.

The Non-Caregiving Spouse

When an adult is caring for a dying parent, the spouse of the caregiver in many cases is involved and supportive of the care provided for an in-law. Sometimes, however, the spouse can be resentful and even jealous of the energy and attention that the caregiving spouse devotes to the dying person. A similar situation can also come about when one parent is caring for a dying child and the other feels neglected or isolated from the intense caregiving relationship. To some extent the caregiver's devotion to the dying person and the spouse's subsequent need to assume more family responsibilities is part of the profound give-and-take that characterizes a successful marriage. As the population ages, it is likely that this caregiving will become one of the more common strains on marriage. Nevertheless, it can create serious conflicts. When they emerge, the hospice social worker can sometimes help to resolve them. If they are serious, more specialized assistance from a marriage counselor might be necessary.

Coping

In the face of caring for someone who is dying, it is very difficult for caregivers to take time out to care for themselves. The frequent advice to take one night off a week and go to a movie or do something for oneself universally went unheeded among those interviewed for this book. Caring for the dying is simply too compelling for caregivers to feel comfortable about going off and enjoying themselves. Many were plagued by an acute sense of lack of time. Would this be the last rainstorm he would see? The last visit by a grandchild? The last time she would hear a favorite record? Or smell a flower? In such an atmosphere, time becomes very precious, and small, ordinary activities take on symbolic significance. Given the meaning caregivers infused into the simplest, everyday occurrences, it was very difficult for them to make time for themselves. Helena Wolf summed up the feelings of most caregivers about this kind of advice:

A lot of people tried to talk to me about how I needed to get distance on the situation and that I needed to not sacrifice my own life and I had to make time for myself even though this was going on. It sounds really good when someone else says this to you, but I think you only do those things if that is your nature; if you have the ability to walk away from something that is totally consuming your life, then you do it in that situation as well. I did do some things. I continued running. I considered it the one sort of salvation that I continued to do.

Taking Breaks

The regular running that Helena managed was similar to the breaks or release that other caregivers found. Sometimes these represented the continuation of regular activities that the caregiver had engaged in prior to undertaking the care of the dying person. In this way the activity served two purposes: it offered respite from the caregiving responsibilities, and it provided a reassuring continuity with the past.

Other caregivers found that short breaks away from the dying person, getting out of the room or house, worked well to defuse tension.

PAT KNOTT: When it got to be too much, I went out on the front porch and sat for a few minutes. Just at those moments when she was grinding her teeth and it wouldn't stop and I would want to scream at her, I would try to leave for a second. I couldn't go for very long, but just walk for a second.

LAURA SWEET: When it got to be too much, I cried a lot, a real lot. Sometimes I'd just go out and walk around the block, go out to a green spot down the way, or would just go on the bed and cry. I cried a lot and talked to my mom on the phone; she was great.

LUCINDA KLEIN: Joyce was verbally abusive. I just kept trying to get on her good side. I yelled back at her sometimes, cried sometimes. One time I left the apartment and sat outside for a few minutes and then went back up. That was actually very effective, but I didn't think of that until quite a while later.

Engaging in a regular activity or hobby that could be done while caring for the person helped some people.

LAURA SWEET: I had plants and flowers and gardening. The one thing that gave me a lot of pleasure—although it sounds silly—was: I had a little box of dirt, four by four, and I grew herbs and flowers on the veranda. That was the only pleasure I got in life, and it gave me a lot of pleasure. I loved to go out there and pick all the weeds and smell the herbs and watch them grow.

PAT KNOTT: I was constantly making things. I did a lot of projects. I think it was something to do if I wasn't doing something specific with Lisa: I needed to keep busy. I didn't have the option of jumping in the car and going off by myself. Keeping busy for me was using my hands. I had a hard time reading and concentrating, but I could do mindless little tasks.

Simply changing the surroundings or concentrating on something other than the caregiving can provide a needed release of tension and a short space in which the caregiver relinquishes the burdens of responsibility. Breaks that are a continuation of past activities—whether they be running, sitting down to dinner, or a monthly bridge game—provide a respite for the caregiver and reestablish some sense of control over and continuity in life. Spontaneous outbursts of anger, frustration, or despair both release tension and provide a brief opportunity for the caregiver to shed some of the responsibility that acute caregiving entails.

Social Support

Chapter 4 described the key role played by social support. As I noted there, being able to talk regularly with another person who is a sympathetic and concerned listener is invaluable for the caregiver. Talking offers caregivers the opportunity to let down, to be emotional, to relieve themselves of the burden of careful, attentive, and responsible caregiving. It also can help caregivers to discuss with supportive others the decisions that must be made. Social support offers a protective social connection demonstrating that, although the caregiver is by necessity isolated and cut off from normal social discourse, the community of friends and neighbors affirms its relationship to her or him.

Mutual support can help alleviate some of the stress that develops between caregivers. When more than one person participates, as in the case of spouses and siblings, they may work well as a team in sharing responsibility yet be too exhausted or strained to find the time to support each other. But they need to try. Other people can help them do this. Such mutual support is a key element in relieving stress, and it allows caregivers to continue. Pat and Don Knott had a friend who watched Lisa so they could take brief walks together.

> PAT KNOTT: I can't say we went out. We were numb; we were just numb. I can't say we went out and had a great time, but we did take these walks. Those kind of breaks were important to our sanity, because we did worry about our sanity. They did a very important thing because they allowed us to be together. Our lives were so coming-and-going the rest of the time, with one person leaving and the other staying with Lisa while the other person did something absolutely essential. The most damning thing about this is that life went on all around you. A lot of things people did allowed us to be together, and for us as a couple it was very important because it was so hard to support each other. When you are just trying to hold yourself together, it is pretty hard to reach out to someone else at that point.

Support Groups and Therapy

In caring for a dying person over an extended period, caregivers may find that the support they receive from family and friends is not adequate. They can turn to more formal sources. In doing so, make sure that the group or therapist is qualified to deal with grief. Most support groups are designed to help people cope with living with a life-threatening disease, not to cope with living with the certainty of imminent death.

Grief therapists specialize in working with dying people and their families. These people can be particularly good at helping the caregiver deal with the dying person's anger and with their own feelings of guilt and inadequacy.

> LAURA SWEET: I had a counselor I went to twice a week. I paid for that myself. It was very important to me to do this, and I always made it to that. I often had to ask someone to be with Tony so I could do it.

> FLORENCE MARTIN: The one saving grace was going to see somebody who was objective and yet worked with patients who were dying and their families. It was the only thing I did for myself, and I really depended on it.

For some diseases there are support groups for the people who have the disease and their caregivers. Several informants said they had tried the cancer support groups and found they were primarily focused on people who were fighting the disease and were not of much use to those who were clearly terminally ill. In contrast, Florence Martin found the group for muscular dystrophy provided valuable information and support. And for Lucinda Klein, the AIDS support group made a significant difference in her ability to cope with caregiving and to handle her anger.

> LUCINDA KLEIN: The only thing I did for myself was my support group. I took a lot of the time of our group. Joyce's problems kept escalating. I didn't follow the advice I got, which was to go out and see a movie, but I talked a lot. The situation was so critical that I just had to go find some help for myself. That's how most of the people got into the group.

In some areas the potential support for people with AIDS and their caregivers is growing, particularly for gays or bisexuals, who tend to come from more integrated, stable, social networks than IV drug users. Thus, although the standard support system—family, neighbors, colleagues, and friends—may not function, it is being replaced, at least partially, by support groups organized specifically for the caregivers of AIDS patients.

Information on support groups or grief therapists can be obtained from a family physician, a hospital or hospice social worker, the local Child and Family Services, or Catholic Social Services (the last two have sliding scales). One can also call the national association for the disease with which the person is afflicted, the National Hospice Organization, or the national office of the Association for Death Education and Counseling (see appendix B for further information).

Laughter

Laughter is wonderful therapy, and almost any opportunity that presents itself for a laugh or smile should be used to the fullest. A hearty laugh will help get rid of negative emotions and tension and will leave the person feeling much better.

The exception is when the laughter is directed at the patient for the "crazy" things demented people sometimes say. As a disease progresses and the body shuts down in anticipation of death, the mind sometimes cannot function clearly or does so only intermittently. People can say some unintentionally funny things when searching for a word they can no longer remember, as when Elizabeth Krolick asked for the "little yellow bunny things" when she wanted an egg to eat. In such situations it is difficult not to laugh, but it is essential to remember that it can be extremely frightening for the dying person, who is often aware that something is seriously wrong with his or her mind. People need to be reassured that it is the disease that has made them say this, and that they are not going crazy. As long as this caution is observed, laughter can be considered a vital resource.

> ANNA KROLICK: I had forgotten to pay the electricity bill, with everything going on, and had to run out and pay it or it would have been disconnected. No matter how hard I tried to argue with the supervisor at the company and say someone was dying, they insisted I come in person and pay it. We had just gotten my mother into the wheelchair and out in the living room when this all happened. I had to rush out before the place closed and left my sister with her little boy and my daughter, and my mother had started screaming that we were trying to kill her. I came back in about twenty minutes and my sister was crying and laughing and the kids and my mother were having a sort of crazy opera of sound. Apparently after initially being afraid of her outburst, the children had decided their grandmother was playing a game with them and they joined in. It was really horrible but also very funny—totally macabre.

Making Life Easier

Caregivers are under extreme strain during this crisis, and it is important that they realize they can't do everything. In some areas, in fact, it may be unwise or even dangerous for them to continue with regular activities if they are too preoccupied with caregiving. Caregivers must impose some limits on the expectations they have of themselves and, if possible, delegate some responsibility to others.

> HELENA WOLF: Driving became almost an impossibility. I finally decided I had to stop driving. I was dangerous; my concentration became so nonexistent that I decided it would not be wise. My husband or brother drove.
>
> I also tried not to have a lot of interactions with people who didn't know what was going on. I couldn't go to the store and have a conversation with a clerk; I would invariably become enraged for no reason. I

wasn't embarrassed. I had no powers of decision making except for what I was actually concentrating on. Going to the grocery store was a disaster. I would walk up and down the aisles and not know what to buy. You think you are concentrating but you are not. I had one preoccupation and that was taking care of my father.

Stan Clark: I let people make some decisions for me because I thought I might not be as rational as I thought I was. I let them make a fuss over me. I realized it was probably not in my best interests or anyone else's for me to try to be in control of everything at that time.

Housework is a key area where others can help the caregiver and where the caregiver can let go and possibly reduce former standards. If having a clean, orderly home is important to the caregiver's sense of order and calm, then it may be worth the money to hire a housekeeper or ask a friend to do this work.

Work

Negotiating more flexible work schedules or leaves of absence was a crucial issue for all the caregivers who worked. The arrangements they made depended on such factors as how much care the dying person required, how much the family relied on the caregiver's income, how long the caregiver had worked at a particular job (the longer the working relationship had existed, the more flexible the employer tended to be), and how long the dying person required care. Helena Wolf took an abrupt leave of absence when she learned of her father's illness:

I was so numb that I just went in to my boss and said that I was taking a leave of absence; my father was dying; good-bye. And I did that with some other people I had responsibilities to—just very abrupt. I don't know if there would have been a better way to do that. I just didn't have a whole lot of patience with convention.

Anna Krolick, who worked as a consultant, was also able to get a leave of absence from her job. Lucille DeMott tried to negotiate a leave. She had recently been hired, and although the company was at first sympathetic, as Jim's illness wore on, it became less and less willing to help her.

Most caregivers could not afford to lose the income caused by a leave of absence. They worked out some combination of more flexible working arrangements supplemented by additional professional or informal support at home. The informal support was most likely when the dying person was not extremely debilitated, as was the case with Alice Clark. Some caregivers who worked felt that their working provided a diversion for them and gave them something to talk with the dying person about; it also provided a valuable break for the caregiver.

> STAN CLARK: Alice and I decided that it was good for me to keep going to work because it brought a different perspective to our lives. We weren't just in our world talking about our problems. We talked about what had happened to me during the day. We weren't so focused on her disease. But I was in touch half a dozen times a day. If something occurred, I would stay home.

> LAURA SWEET: Tony would look forward to my coming home because I had this job and hated my boss. I would come home and bitch to him, and I think he liked that. He would get into bitching with me and talking about what had happened during the day. I am glad I did that because I couldn't have gone out and had fun by myself, and I really needed to get away sometimes.

When a caregiver is working, assuming the responsibility for a dying person at home will require at least some—if not significant—adjustment in workload and flexibility in attendance. This may also be the case for other members of the family who are providing vital support. Most caregivers were moved by the sensitivity or willingness to be flexible demonstrated by their employers and fellow workers.

> PAT KNOTT: Don's firm had just opened an office in town, and they were extremely accommodating. The people who could do this reassigned Don's clients and gave him some in our town so he could work here instead of having to commute. He was just told, "You don't have these clients, go work in your hometown."

Employers, especially those in small businesses, are limited in the arrangements they can make. Caregivers need to consider the limits of their work situation as well as their need for income when they make the decision to care for someone at home. As we saw in chapter 2, it is rare that professional support can substitute for the presence of a caregiver. If the dying person requires full-time care—

and many do—dependable informal support must be found, or the employed caregiver must consider either taking a leave of absence or placing the dying person in a hospital or nursing home.

Spiritual Support

In the face of the often excruciating demands of caregiving, several people turned to spiritual support to help them sustain their efforts and to give them the strength to continue. Importantly, spiritual support provided some people with a way of explaining the death and helped them maintain a sense of continuity and control in their lives. Sometimes they had clergy visit the home, sometimes they visited a place of worship, or they prayed on their own.

> HELEN WRIGHT: It's the kind of space that—you find the strength because you have to have it. I think my constant prayer was "Don't let me be afraid and don't let me be anxious and just be with what is; be there, be here for whatever needs to be done." So I was pretty positive. Only occasionally would I just feel, sort of, I wasn't really very sad because you just can't let it in, you just have to keep everything up.

What Enabled Caregivers to Care and What It Meant to Them

All of the caregivers in this study said they were frequently asked how they could do what they did. Although most said clearly that this was *not* something that everyone should attempt, they did not see themselves as special. Some attributed their ability to do this to the models their parents had set for them.

> PAT KNOTT: I had the advantage of watching my father go through the process and being extremely determined that my mother would stay at home. I have had great admiration for my father in the way he handled that process.

> LAURA SWEET: My mother was a good mother, and I think I probably carry some of her traits in that way; taking care of other people is a learned behavior.

Others felt that their past experience in caring for the dying—either as family members or in their professional lives—prepared them.

BONNIE STEINER: It's never been difficult for me to talk to people who were dying. I always could do that with patients. They would pour out their guts to me. I had often thought that if I could do that in my life, I would like to have a job in a hospital where that is what I did—have a lab coat on and go around and talk to people about death.

LUCILLE DEMOTT: I had an idea: I had previously had to deal with grief and dying in the workplace. I had to contact bereaved families and I would visit terminally ill patients. My aunt died at home and my brother had been killed. I felt I had some knowledge of death, more than many people. My idea was that the environment we ought to make around Jim should be one of love and help.

Past experience did not always prepare people for the intensity of emotions one experiences in caring for a dying person. In this study, three physicians participated informally, as family members or as friends, in providing care for the dying person. They all said that neither their training nor their practice had prepared them for the intensity or complexity of this caregiving. Pat Knott, a nurse, was very aware of the difference between caring for a family member and caring for a patient:

> It didn't matter what you had done before because when you are doing it for your own family member, it is somehow different. It makes you realize how much you detach yourself as a caregiver in a hospital. I learned that with my mom. My father asked me to do the suctioning, and I found myself in tears doing her suctioning because she would choke and have difficulty breathing. I had suctioned I can't tell you how many people. I could always before say, "It will just be another minute, just hold on." But I couldn't say that with my mother.
> And somehow when you see your own child obviously in pain, you can't detach yourself. Even though as a nurse, I thought I wasn't a detached nurse, I realized I was. The reason was probably because if you have an emotional attachment to every patient, you wouldn't survive. I couldn't detach myself. The detachment wasn't there.

The familiarity with death which some caregivers had did not reduce the intensity of the experience. It did, however, help them know what to expect, which left them without fear of the death itself.

Some caregivers attributed their ability to care for the dying person simply to their love for that person.

LUCINDA KLEIN: I wanted her home because I really loved her and because it was really helpful to take care of her. The thought of her being someplace where I couldn't readily get to see her. . . . I really did want the responsibility. I never thought that I was someone—well, I never had any experience in taking care of people in this way. I don't have any younger siblings; my parents are in good health. My response kind of surprised me. But once she got sick, it was all that I cared about doing, taking care of her. I never resented spending all that time at the hospital or home with her. I didn't find it distressing or ugly that I was dressing her bedsores or that I was wiping her after she urinated. I just didn't. Those were things that I thought would've bothered me, and they just really didn't at all. I was really glad to be able to do it.

Others attributed their ability to care to aspects of their personality.

STAN CLARK: It goes back to the question about how I could do this. We were so much in touch that I didn't have a lot of baggage or resentment about her behavior, and at the same time we were talking together enough that I felt that I understood what she wanted and all that.

A strong religious faith sustained others in their roles as caregivers.

HELEN WRIGHT: I was with my mother when she died, the last few days. It had been a very good experience. And I was with my grandfather when he died, and it was very positive; the family was very positive. There was a great deal of faith that there was a passing over into another life, and so I didn't feel that it was the end, and that made a difference. It made a lot of difference.

Many caregivers felt that all the trouble, stress, and exhaustion they experienced were worth it because of the intimacy they achieved with the dying person and because they were assured they had helped provide the best possible death.

JOE STEAD: I think I did a hell of a lot better job than they did in the hospital because I was with her. Whatever she wanted, if it was possible to do for her, I did it. Made no difference what it was. No way I would have put her back in the hospital. That was because she was mine and I wanted to see that she was taken care of, and she wanted to be here and she wanted to be with her family and her family with her.

LUCINDA KLEIN: The understanding which we came to about our relationship in the last few weeks before she died was really remarkable. That was the best part about what I did. I know that she really appreciated that I didn't leave, that I was there all the time, that I kept coming to the hospital, that I kept coming home after work and I had energy for her. That I kept doing the laundry, which was a lot, and the shopping. She would say that she knew that this was a lot. I was glad that I had it in me. It was a surprise because I realized my parents had never done something like this; they never went through this kind of caregiving. It is good to know you can do this.

Some, however, felt that the strain had been too much and vowed never to do this again.

FLORENCE MARTIN: I have been through it with a father, a mother, and a husband. I am just not interested in doing it again. I definitely have a great fear of, if I did remarry again, of having to take care of another person until they died. I just want to take care of me for a change.

Caring for a dying person at home is one of the most significant and meaningful, as well as difficult, tasks anyone can undertake. The responsibility for making it work ultimately lies with the caregiver. This fact in the end, in and of itself, should deter those who are not physically strong enough and those who are uncomfortable with assuming responsibility or exercising authority from attempting home death. Like the long-distance runner I spoke of earlier, caregivers must attend to their own well-being—physical and emotional—to ensure that they can continue to function effectively for the dying person's sake as well as their own.

To see the dying person through until death or until it is agreed that the patient should be placed in a hospital or nursing home provides the caregiver with an immense sense of accomplishment. This was a solace for many in coping with their grief. But because the stress is substantial, the caregivers must attend to themselves both to ensure the success of caregiving and to avoid impeding the renewal and regeneration that must take place after a death occurs.

CHAPTER SIX

Demystifying Death

Americans—those in their fifties and younger—have had little experience in caring for the dying or in seeing a person die. The prospect of having someone die at home, of being present at the actual death, can be very frightening. The fear goes beyond the apprehension and grief associated with awaiting the death of a loved one. It is the fear of the unknown. Will the death be painful? Will it be grotesque? How will I know the person is actually dying or even dead? What will happen afterward? These fears, many of which are nameless, some of which are very concrete ("I didn't want my mother to die in Susan's room; I was afraid she could never sleep there after that"), can lead caregivers to hospitalize or institutionalize a patient on the verge of death. Such transfers are warranted when the caregiver is completely burned out and there is no replacement caregiver: the welfare of both caregiver and dying person is at stake. They are also appropriate in cases where there is uncontrolled pain. Many such transfers, however, are due to inadequate preparation of the caregiver and to insufficient professional support for the caregiver and dying person.

The purpose of this chapter is to present the caregivers' accounts of the deaths they participated in, to illustrate how death occurs. Death is not a supernatural occurrence but a profoundly natural one. It may not be as easy as the overly optimistic description offered by many physicians that "the patient will slip into a coma and die quietly," but neither is it as intimidating as the popularized depictions of death in television and movies. This chapter is designed to demystify death and thus to reduce the apprehension that caregivers such as Laura Sweet felt:

> Toward the end when he was doing funny breathing, probably a lot of it was my own imagination and paranoia and heightened sense of aware-

ness, but I really felt that he was going to die any time and I would wake up with a cold, stiff body next to me. I didn't know anything about death. I was afraid I was going to see a ghost and it was going to be scary. I had a flashlight and wouldn't go to the bathroom in the dark. I had to have the flashlight with me, and it was only six feet from the bedroom. I was scared he was going to die in bed.

Maybe it was too many movies. I thought he was going to take these gasping last breaths and just expire and this filmy white substance would—this spirit would come out of him. I thought I would feel his presence leaving, maybe a cold chill.

I was sort of disappointed when he actually died. It was after five hours of cleaning all this shit up that was coming out of him. I said, "Whew, we can finally go to sleep now that he is resting peacefully," and I looked at him and "Wait a minute he doesn't look like he is breathing." I went over and he wasn't. I had entirely missed the actual death. It wasn't what I was expecting. I was expecting more of a Hollywood type of event. I don't know if other people feel differently. I have read something about death and have read that some people feel a presence in the room. That did not happen to me.

Caregivers are under enough pressure without having to suffer from exaggerated fears, fears that can be allayed with information, preparation, and adequate professional support.

Signs of Approaching Death

The following is a list of the signs of approaching death and suggestions for the caregiver. Not all the signs will appear at the same time, and some may never appear:

- Sensation and the ability to move, as well as reflexes, are lost. This happens first in the legs and moves to the arms. To prevent pressure on the skin, turn the person frequently; this will also make him or her more comfortable.
- The arms and legs may become cool and appear darker in color as a result of decreased circulation. A light blanket will make the patient more comfortable. Do not use an electric blanket.
- The amount of time spent sleeping will increase, and the person will be difficult to arouse. The presence of someone nearby will be reassuring, even though the dying person may appear to be unaware of the presence.

- The patient may become confused about time or place or be unable to recognize close friends or family members. Frequently mention the time and day and who is in the room by name. This will be reassuring. Explaining that this is the result of the disease process and that the person is not going crazy will also help.
- As sight fails, the dying person should be turned on the side toward the light. The room should be well lit and the people in the room should be at the head of the bed because of the person's decreasing ability to see.
- The sense of hearing remains acute until death. *Never assume that the dying person cannot hear what is being said.*
- The dying person may lose control of urine and bowel. Keep the patient on a draw sheet with an underpad made for incontinence. As death nears, urine output may cease or change color.
- Oral secretions may increase and collect in the back of the throat. Elevate the head of the bed and consult the nurse.
- Restlessness, pulling on linen, having visions of people or things, can occur. Make sure that someone remains with the person and provides reassurance.
- The need for food and drink will decrease. Keep the mouth moist by giving ice chips or, if the person is unable to swallow, wipe the tongue with olive oil. *Do not force food or drink.*
- When death is near, there may be irregular breathing with a rattle in the throat and periods of no breathing. The person may seem relaxed and without pain during this time.

When death has occurred:

- There is no breathing.
- There is no heartbeat (take a pulse and count respirations every fifteen minutes until no vital signs can be obtained).
- The eyelids are open.
- The eyes are fixed on a certain spot.
- The jaw is relaxed and the mouth slightly open.

Immediately after Death

Emergency Medical Services (EMS)

For many when the death occurs, a kind of panic can set in and there is a strong impulse to call the **Emergency Medical Service (EMS)**.

Don't do this. When an EMS team arrives, the members assume authority in the situation. If they decide to try to revive the person, they have this right regardless of what the family or even the attending hospice nurse wants. Many EMS personnel can recognize that a death is planned and that this is simply an occasion in which the caregiver needs to be reassured and calmed down. Others will insist on doing an **electrocardiogram** and attempting CPR. If they are successful in their attempt, they will transport the dying person to the hospital, where he or she will be placed on life support. Getting someone disconnected from these systems then is extremely difficult, as many lawsuits testify.

Having a hospice nurse in attendance should avoid the problem because hospice personnel can reassure the family and dissuade them from calling the EMS. Call the hospice team if they are not already present. If there is no professional in the home to reassure the family, hospices recommend that caregivers not call EMS until the body is cold. Usually this precaution will prevent the EMS from any attempt at resuscitation. Unfortunately, in some cases the EMS will attempt to revive the person anyway—much to the horror and anguish of the family members.

In some states it is possible to avoid unwanted resuscitation by having the physician, with the dying person's approval (or the family's, if the person is no longer competent), write a **"Do not resuscitate" (DNR)** order, which can be posted above the bed. The order indicates that the dying person or someone competent to make a decision for her or him does not want the person to be resuscitated should a life-threatening event occur. (See appendix D for examples of a letter requesting a physician to do this, and of a physician's letter.)

In some states the physician can sign the death certificate in advance when the patient is diagnosed as terminally ill, and this can be presented to the EMS, or to the funeral director if funeral arrangements have already been made. Other states allow nurses to pronounce death. This is probably the best solution. It permits the nurse to proceed to help the family arrange for the funeral and have the body transported directly to the funeral home, completely avoiding the potential problems of dealing with the EMS.

Because state laws differ with respect to the use of DNR orders and persons allowed to pronounce death, it is best to find out what the law in your particular state is by asking the hospice nurse or doctor or by calling a funeral home. Thinking this through in advance will help forestall the panicked impulse to call EMS.

Removing the Body

Much of the appeal of a home death, as I have repeatedly stated, lies in the freedom to decide how the dying person will spend the last part of his or her life. In the home, the regulations, restrictions, and interference of institutional authorities can be avoided as well. Home death allows individuals to continue to exercise a degree of control over their lives. It is appropriate for caregivers to extend this control to the decision of when to remove the body.

As will become clear in the following accounts, many chose to have the body remain in the home for several hours, sometimes as many as ten, after the death. The caregivers who did this clearly felt that the immediate removal of the body, which is customary in American funerary practice, was far too soon. They were not yet reconciled to the separation. During the hours in which the body remained in the home, these people gradually came to separate themselves from it. They all eventually felt that it was time for the body to leave and "time to get on with the next stage." In other words, the same caregivers who were opposed to removing the body soon after death accepted this move several hours later.

Many of the caregivers who had the body remain in the home held an informal wake in which family and friends gathered to say good-bye to the deceased and to reminisce about the person's life and about the dying process. Caregivers remarked that the social contact at this time was particularly helpful to them.

Children

The following accounts of people's deaths provide different examples of the degree to which children were involved in the dying process and in seeing the body after death. Children from a very young age, if given the opportunity, are able to make choices about both. Whenever possible, their wishes should be respected. It is natural that a child might be curious to see the dead person; this is not idle curiosity, nor are children likely to take inappropriate advantage of the situation. All the children discussed here who were given the opportunity to choose, and who chose to see the body, were serious and respectful in its presence.

Whether children wish to see the dying person or the body or not, they will have many, many questions about what is happening and what it means. Adults should offer numerous opportunities for children to talk and to ask questions. It is possible that they will not do this immediately, perhaps sensing that an adult is too upset to talk about the death. At some point, however, children will want to talk or should be encouraged to talk, and adults should try to be open to these inquiries despite the pain they may cause. If children are in school or preschool, their teachers should be informed of what is happening at home. It is possible that children in such a stressful situation will alter their behavior, and it is important that the teachers understand the reason for the change.

Suicide

Suicide was considered by four of the patients in this book; one actually took her own life. Suicide is always an option for the terminally ill person—indeed, it is an option for everyone—but several things relating to the care the person is receiving could influence the decision and should be considered.

1. If uncontrolled pain is the reason for considering suicide, have the pain evaluated by a hospice physician and nurse. If one hospice program cannot control the pain, try another. Pain control should be possible to achieve with the help of an appropriately trained professional. In cases of uncontrolled pain, the person can be hospitalized, and pain can be alleviated in the hospital setting.
2. If the desire is to spare the family the burden of caregiving, allow family members to express themselves about this. They may wish to provide care for the dying person in recognition of their love for that person. Suicide deprives them of this. With one exception, all the caregivers interviewed here found caring for the dying one of the most significant accomplishments in their lives.
3. Seek professional counseling. The dying person may be depressed and afraid. Professional counseling may help the patient deal with these emotions and go on to live out the rest of his or her life. Clergy who have experience in counseling the dying can be especially helpful in this respect.

4. Sometimes people contemplate suicide because they feel the disease forces them to lose all control over their lives. Suicide is seen as a way of reestablishing control. For this reason the contemplation of and preparation for suicide can have a calming and healing effect. Having regained the sense of control over life which the decision to end life can create, many people then decide against suicide. Their decision remains as an option that gives them strength to face an uncertain future. Professional counseling should be used here also, but the caregiver and dying person need to be aware that a professional response may be positive or negative to a potential suicide. The counselor may be helpful in working this issue through and realize that such an approach to a terminal illness can be positive, or may feel obliged to try to have the person committed as a danger to himself or herself. In selecting a counselor it is important to find someone with considerable experience in working with the dying.

5. If the person remains intent on suicide, information is available from the Hemlock Society which describes how to kill oneself without prescription drugs. A serious problem for many potential suicides is failure that permanently maims, resulting in hospitalization for the remainder of the person's life. Following the Hemlock Society methods will ensure that death results. (See appendix B for more information.)

6. Physician-assisted suicide is an option that has received considerable public attention due to the efforts of Dr. Jack Kevorkian. In many cases the desire for physician-assisted suicide is the result of intractable pain, depression, or both. The steps listed above can be followed to help resolve the problems underlying the suicide wish. If these steps fail, or if the wish persists despite them, individual state laws need to be consulted to determine whether physician-assisted suicide is legal in a particular state, under what circumstances, and what safeguards are in place to prevent inappropriate use of this procedure. Identifying a physician willing to supervise the death may be an additional challenge.

Some Who Died at Home

Alice Clark

STAN CLARK: She had asked her sister to handle her funeral. We had gone to the funeral parlor to see the husband of a friend of mine who died of a heart attack. We went so we could see what that was like, and it reassured her that she didn't want any part of that. She didn't want any part of being on display. I thought maybe she wanted her sister to arrange the funeral because she would do a jazzy scene. But later I realized it was another one of her sensitivities—that she wanted to make sure that someone besides me had some responsibility.

The bunch of people who had been helping knew she was having trouble and came around the day before she died and the day she died. Almost everyone that did anything with her was there. I wanted them to be there. There were probably twelve people there when Alice died. Whoever wasn't there came over soon after. These people later said this was the most significant thing in their lives, a very helpful thing for them. Their admiration for Alice for her courage, for her sensitivity to them, for her nobility as a social human being, was such that I have these unbelievable letters from these people.

A friend of ours, a controlled, objective physician, came about three hours before Alice died to say good-bye. She said, "I have never done this before." She was crying. "Is it all right with you if I do it? I have to say good-bye to her." So she went in. At this time Alice's speech was hard to understand. But I heard it from the other room. Alice pleaded. Sue was telling her how much she meant to her, what a heroic person and sensitive person she was, and how it mattered to her to have known her.

Alice kept her concern about others' well-being and concerns. The Blacks came to visit that last afternoon, and Alice said to Judy, who had just come back from a job interview, "Did you get a job?" Another dear friend of mine who had been helping me came in, and Alice said something about her being a dear friend. She stayed like herself—even close to death. She was always so considerate, but this quality was also a source of distraction. It helped her to focus on other people. Maybe you don't need to be distracted but I guess that is part of my view of the whole thing. If you are scared, you handle it by focusing on something else, a distraction.

The evening, twenty-four hours before she died, Alice was feeling really bad and struggling on her own. Our regular nurse had this idea to have the kids look at old family pictures, and Alice was doing that with them, and saying, "Do you remember this?" I was kind of there with her and doing deep breathing, and the rest of the family was sitting around and talking about photographs and saying, "Remember how we used to do this," and then they would say something to Alice about it. Part of it she got and part of it she didn't, because she was in real tough shape. Laughing at the photos and talking about the good or funny times we had had was particularly helpful for the kids at that time.

She rallied the morning she died. That was when she said, "I was all ready last night; now what do I have to do?" Her sister came, and Alice complimented her on how gorgeous she looked. Then she started to get distressed, and I said, "Why don't you do some golf with Beth?" Her sister was a superb golfer. That had been an early distraction. So she started pretending to play the club course. "I will take a nine iron and go so many yards" and Beth joined her in the pretend game. Alice was absolutely alert. Then she started having difficulty in breathing and said she'd better return to the club house. Her breathing became really labored about 4 P.M.

I would lie on the bed with her on the afternoon of the day that she died and do the breathing exercises and try to do some holding off of the coldness and the terrible sweats that she had. It didn't seem right for her to be alone. I did a lot of the breathing routine we had for panic reduction. I remember I was going to the door with someone and she called me and it was one of those panic times.

When she died her two sisters and my three kids and I were all immediately there at the bedside; probably another ten people were there in the living room and dining room area.

I started to say, "What are you doing?" to the nurse. The other nurse who was there then was moving the TV away—moving everything away so we could stand by the bed. She started telling my sister-in-law she had to be there by the bed and my sister-in-law said, "I don't want to be there." In the last few minutes of life Alice was still indicating the need for a bedpan because she had a sensation of losing her bowel control. And she had me hold onto her.

The doctor whom we both cared about was not there. He was attending a big dinner party, something unusual. Now I know that he wouldn't have cared that he had a dinner party going or not; he would have liked to be there when Alice died. He was really upset at not being there, and he was very angry at not having been called so he could give his direction for more morphine because Alice was soaking wet, just pouring sweat water off her. She had difficulty just breathing. She couldn't talk. I didn't want her to go, so I wasn't thinking. I got so angry at that nurse I said, "Listen, I am going to call the doctor," and the nurse said, "I just did." Before that she had been saying, "I don't think we should disturb the doctor." The doctor had been so personally involved with Alice's care that he became visibly upset about her dying.

I may not have given Alice enough opportunity to talk about dying. We both did a kind of protection thing against that. I mean, I don't feel horrible; she did talk about that some. I think once having been through the entire experience, I would have done more straight-out stuff from the very beginning. I think your not talking about that may make the person feel they cannot talk about it. She told me everything she was feeling but not if she was scared—she didn't directly say it, like, "My God, what is going to happen? How do you suppose death is going to occur? I am scared about the final pain." I didn't talk to her about stuff like that, which I think I might have since she was talkable. I don't know if that would have made a difference.

There is a whole big difference in taking care of someone like that who is talking to you up until the last minute. I can't imagine you would have the same kind of participation by friends in the situation when the patient is mentally incapacitated, blind, or deaf. I can't imagine I would have asked people in the same way to come and take care of her if it had been really nursing or intimate custodial care.

Jim DeMott

LUCILLE DeMOTT: The physician thought two weeks earlier—this was when Philip left—that Jim was dying. Throughout these several months of the disease process, Jim was a unique human being in terms of always deciding to live, to fight the battle for life. So I think that he fought one more battle but this time it was too much. He was unable to speak and the other systems were shutting down and he was completely immobile at this time. The physician thought his death could occur at any time.

I could see all the changes in his body and hear the changes in his breathing pattern. We still had a sexual relationship when he was hobbling across the room on his walker. Then there came a time when he just didn't want that anymore but he wanted touching. There were a lot of things going on where you could see his body shut down; you could see it occur.

No one told me about the physiology of dying until he was dying.

The hospice administrator gave me some very valuable information about three months before his death—that we did not have to have Jim removed from the house immediately after he had died. In our state we had twenty-four hours. Hospice had connected me with a mortician who had some kind of hospice philosophy, so that they were willing to pick up the body when the family was ready. That was very useful information to have ahead of time. I knew that, because he had been in the home terminally ill, the physician could sign the death certificate ahead of time according to state law. The physician had signed the death certificate about two weeks before Jim died and told me it was all signed in case he wasn't available when the death occurred so we could call the mortician when we wanted.

I knew he was actually dying because of his breathing pattern. I had heard breathing problems that night as I had heard them many times before in the hospital with Jim when he almost died. The respiratory change awoke me and I already knew the swallowing response had just about disappeared and that he had little awake time.

I called the VNA [Visiting Nurse Association] because he obviously had pain. He had morphine and we were increasing it. The VNA nurse had come to the house. We were talking about what to do to help him, and she told me then that he was in fact dying. She described the dying process and said that he would die in the next few hours. We talked about what to do and she recommended unobstructing the bowels, which we did and which he was alert for despite all the morphine. His eyes were giving an expression of horror; it must have been a very painful thing. It was a hard decision: should you relieve some pain at that time or should you just give him more morphine? I don't know what was the right decision. The nurse didn't know how long he might live and she knew the bowel was very, very uncomfortable and causing a lot of pain. He didn't like that at all.

Afterwards she and I bathed him and made him as comfortable as possible. As he slept, she described (out of the room) what was going on and what I could expect. She said that she was leaving and that I could call if I wanted to but I didn't have to. We went back into the room and found him in the process of dying. The blood was not circulating in his lower limbs anymore, which I didn't notice, interestingly enough. His face was fine, and she pointed out to me the areas where the blood was not circulating. He appeared to be sleeping. Then he opened his eyes and smiled and did his version of talking. At the time he did that, his limbs were blue up to the joints; it was incredible. She said she had never seen anything like it. He died very soon after. The kids chose not to be there. They came in right after.

We kept him at home ten hours or longer. I hadn't planned for it to be that long, but a friend wanted to see him and had trouble getting there. So I just decided it was O.K. for him to be there. It turned out to be nice. I had decided I wanted to be the one to do the last things with his physical being and I couldn't do that right away. I just sobbed and sobbed and dealt with the kids. The kids were not good; none of us were good. We were all real sad and upset. We didn't feel relief at all, just real sadness and loneliness.

As the day went on friends came in to say good-bye, and we ended up having a little backyard party in the evening. The kids were a part of this and we were doing a lot of remembrances of Jim. It was kind of like an old-fashioned wake. We remembered some of the humor of the funny situations there had been during his care when he had giggled; and there was just a real nice camaraderie over the whole thing. A time came when it felt right to call the mortician and get on with the next steps.

I had gone to give my last good-bye, and the mortician suggested I probably would want to leave because they put the body in a body bag. The have to put the body on a gurney and down the stairs, and it doesn't always work very smoothly. I had done the last care of his physical body. I had him in the pajamas I wanted him to be in and all of that felt good; there was something very loving and touching about all of that. You know how frequently people say it is cold and awful: it isn't like that at all. It was very pleasant, warm, loving kind of thing that felt very natural. I felt love and O.K.; but seeing the body in a body bag did not feel good. I saw it. That was not a good thing to do and I sure wouldn't let a kid see that.

It helped my children a lot to see their father. But who has proof of those things? Philip was always opting in or out of the process on the basis of discussions and what he could see. If a kid is at all old enough, that is a good way to make the decision. He was young—only seven. In the end he opted to be there. I had awakened him that morning and told him that it was going to happen pretty soon and that he could come in and say good-bye to his dad. Both children did that, but they didn't want to be in the room right when he died. They did come into the room, and they did see him, and they did touch him, too. We made it all work as if everyone did this. It didn't seem like something different.

I was not sure that children should deal with seeing the body leave. They had said their good-byes. I didn't really know what to expect. I had adults keeping the kids away so they wouldn't see the body leaving the house. We kept them out of that whole part of the house. They never even saw the mortician. For us that was the appropriate kind of dividing line.

Lisa Knott

PAT KNOTT: I was afraid of dying in the sense that I worried about how it might happen, and I remember discussing it with her oncologist. Would she—how might she die? Would she bleed to death? What were the possibilities, because I wanted to be prepared for what might happen and to then know what we were going to do.

I think by that first week there was this part of us that wanted to have her die because we felt that at that point it was inevitable. There was this part of us that almost just said "die" then; and there was this other part that still bargained and wished it could be different. I think I knew she was going to die and I knew somehow I would go through that in the same way I had gone through the rest of it. I never had any inclination to run her to the hospital at any time. That was part of saying to this oncologist, "What are the possibilities? Might she die quietly in her sleep? Is she going to bleed to death? Is she going to get a terrible infection? Is she going to be debilitated?" That was part of getting ready for whatever was going to happen.

As it happened, her condition had really changed and her breathing had become much slower. This had happened over a period of twenty-four hours. In fact, we were thinking of going out for a walk and a friend had come over and we were sitting on the couch talking to her and she had just come. It was Saturday. Don said, "Her breathing has just gotten much slower." We sat on the bed with her and I picked her up and within ten minutes she died. She—her breath just went slower and slower. It was like she was sleeping. Although we had noticed a difference in her, we obviously wouldn't have been thinking about going out for a walk if we had thought that right at that moment it was really going to change.

Don called her doctor and the funeral director. We had talked to him earlier, which is a very ghoulish, funny feeling. Then we called a minister, a friend, who came over, and that night some friends came over. The friend who orchestrated everything, who set up the visitors—they came over that night. Actually that first night we decided to go to the park. We just went out there. I have no idea why we went out there. We were just driving and we went out there and we walked around there for awhile. There weren't too many people. Then we came home and some friends came over and just sat and talked. The funeral home came within a couple of hours.

I don't remember feeling afraid of her death. I remember sitting on the bed after she died and stroking her head and talking to her and feeling almost relieved for her. Because I had gone through the experience with my mom, I wasn't fearful.

My mom died at home and I was with her when she died. I think that just made a huge difference. I just knew that I wanted to be at home and I wanted her to be at home. My mother had been very definite about not wanting to go to the hospital. Over a period of months she reinforced it with us. She said, "I want to be here, please don't take me to the hospital." We had been with her. I think that I had that relatively recent experience and that made a big difference. Another thing that made a difference was being a health care professional, and seeing people come into the hospital who ended up on respirators, who ended up living when it wasn't at all what their family had wanted to happen for them. I have seen that many, many times, so I think that was probably there too, knowing that I didn't want to be a person who landed in the ER [emergency room] and had all these things done to me at that point. I didn't want that for Lisa. My mother knew she didn't want that for herself.

Elizabeth Krolick

ANNA KROLICK: The Friday before she died, I had actually gone to a meeting at work, something I hadn't done all month. When I came home, we had one of the best discussions we had had since she came home. She appeared very clear; her speech was clear; she asked to see my daughter, who uncharacteristically wouldn't talk with her. Mother had been bad the day before, refusing all food and then the aide came again on Friday and she perked up. She said she thought the aide, whom she had become very attached to, had abandoned her. She drank a lot of fluids and seemed really fine.

That night she began complaining that her mouth really hurt her and she couldn't swallow. We gave her the first Dilaudid suppository and she seemed to sleep. Next morning about seven, she couldn't swallow and began this continual attempt to cough something up, to clear her throat. She seemed very uncomfortable and asked for a pain pill, which was very unusual: she almost never asked for a pain pill. We gave her Dilaudid again because she couldn't take anything by mouth. We called the hospital and they said she might have a film in her throat. She fell asleep with the Dilaudid, and the aide was able to clean out her mouth and her eyes. At this point her eyes were clouded over with pus but she wouldn't let us touch them except for putting a wet cloth on them.

I think we tried to get my sister at this point and couldn't reach her. As it turned out, she had gone to the cottage and not told us. My brother and daughter and I went shopping and got the urn for my mother—that was weird—and had breakfast. When we got back about eleven-thirty— and the aide was really alarmed. Mother seemed to be choking a lot, and was clearly distressed. She just looked out the window, hanging onto the side of the bed, trying to breathe. My husband had already called the nurse and she came soon after we got back. The nurse said things were much worse, which we could clearly see, and that she wouldn't last many more days because she could no longer take any fluids except when we would drop water on the gauze over her mouth, which she always removed. Eric decided to postpone his departure till Monday morning.

I had a strong feeling that Mother was thinking about her father, whom she watched choke to death with lung cancer. We agreed to increase the Dilaudid. The nurse left and kept calling. A friend had taken my daughter Nancy [three years old] for the day and brought her back, and her asthma was really bad. She was also exhausted, so I put her to bed and kept checking her breathing. David left to get some sleep at a friend's apartment, and my brother went to bed so he could take the night shift. Nancy's breathing kept getting worse and about twelve-thirty I decided to take her to the ER. I called my neighbor and asked her to help my brother if he needed it. She said she would, then left her answering machine on, which prevented Eric from reaching her. I called my sister-in-law, a physician, and found out how much more medication we could give, then I woke up Eric and we increased her pain medication and turned her. I called the nurse and told her I was leaving for the hospital and that Eric might need help.

I kept calling Eric from the hospital and Mother was getting worse. He thought she had a stroke because she started holding one side of her face and seemed to be in more pain. I tried to explain what was happening to the ER docs, but their only response was to suggest I hospitalize my mother. They insisted my daughter be admitted. Eric called the nurse about 4 A.M. and she came and helped him until David arrived at 5:30. He stayed with Mother until 11, then he came to the hospital to relieve me and stay with our daughter.

When I got home, I could see she was much worse. We had a new regime of increased and more frequent pain meds, and we had to wipe her mouth out with olive oil every half-hour. I had breakfast and took a nap. Mother's best friend came over and sat with her while we slept. I got up and the friend went to go shopping. Eric was up and we kept trying to reach our sister. Mother was continually getting worse, but very alert.

This whole thing went very fast and was very intense. Eric wanted to take a nap and so I had my neighbor come over so I wouldn't be alone. We went in and gave Mother a massage and more medication and turned her. She seemed to be in a lot of pain, and I called my sister-in-law to see if I could increase the pain meds again. She didn't resist being turned and when I asked if she wanted more medication, she nodded, "Yes." I began going into her room every fifteen minutes to put oil on her tongue. It was too horrible to be in there and she seemed very concentrated on herself and not really wanting us there; it was a very strong feeling we had; but it was also so, so hard because she seemed to be suffering and we couldn't do anything to help her except brush her tongue with oil and the inside of her mouth. She continued to hold the side of the bed. And of course we had no idea she was actually dying. The nurse had said a couple of days, so that was what we thought.

Eric got up and sat with us making lists of who would be here when. He was considering not leaving if Mother continued to be that bad, and I was very relieved. We also decided to call our sister and tell her to come, but we still couldn't find her, so we had [one of her neighbors] put notes on her door. Finally we found her at the cottage and she tried to get a plane here. Eric went to check on Mother and called me. I knew the minute I heard his voice that she had died.

Eric started sobbing and we called my neighbor who was there and was a doctor. She came in and confirmed that Mother was dead. She tried to put her hands in a peaceful manner—Mother had been holding on to the bed railing when she died—and to close her eyes, but they kept opening. We hugged her and held her hands. I called our pediatrician to help me get my daughter out of the hospital. My neighbor went with me to get her, and her husband came over so Eric wouldn't be alone. Mother's friend came back with the groceries and the nurse arrived. Another friend who had helped take care of her came over. The funeral people came, but David told them to go away, we weren't ready to have her go. The nurse gave her a rose to put in her arms.

Different people came over and went in and said good-bye and held her hands, which were gradually getting colder and stiffer. My daughter went in to say good-bye but wouldn't touch her even though I held

Mother's hand and kissed her. We had dinner and then she had to go back to the hospital, which she really didn't want to do. David went with her and spent the night.

Mother's friend and another friend and Eric and I sat up and drank wine and talked about Mother and about what taking care of her had been like. Finally the funeral home called saying they had to pick her up or pay overtime. Eric and Mother's friend and I went into her room and stayed until they came. Then we stood together and did a soft shoe dance while they carried her out. I am sure they thought we were crazy but I know she would have loved it. It was a kind of tribute to her, to the kind of person she was.

Al Martin

FLORENCE MARTIN: When his children were here at Christmas, he told them all good-bye. He told them all differently. The oldest boy sobbed. The next boy he told good-bye, but the third son is the one who had done the most for him and had always done the most for him, and he wouldn't even talk to him. It was very strange. But he denied death until the last four days. I think—I don't know if he died from too much carbon dioxide. He got so he could not exhale, so a lot of the time he got so he did not know what was going on.

I think my husband, once he saw his sister, he was ready to die. He didn't fight as much. He wanted a shower every day no matter how much it tired him out; everything had to be just so. Then he got so as he didn't care type of thing. He just was ready.

I almost felt that he had almost died the week before he died. I had gone to the store, and this other lady was here, and he looked like he was sleeping. He had trouble with his eyes. His eyes would roll up in his head. So for two months I never knew whether he was dead or not when I got up. Here was this man with his eyes rolled up and he would breathe so softly you couldn't tell whether he was breathing or not. She said all of a sudden he got this terrible look on his face—and just awful—and she screamed at him and she had to do it three or four times and he finally woke up, and she asked him some questions: he couldn't talk. She asked him, had he been going down a tunnel and he said yes, which I guess is one of the things that people who have stopped breathing and been brought back—this happens to them. I don't know. But I still wonder if he wouldn't have died the week before if she hadn't noticed this was happening to him.

He died in his sleep. I had been up with him to two in the morning.

From Friday on, we knew he was dying. Evidently he knew that he was dying, because the lady came on Sunday—it was her birthday—and she said, "You aren't going to die on my birthday, are you?" and he shook his head, "no." And she said, "I'll see you tomorrow morning," and he shook his head, "no." We had a really bad storm and I was in the room with him, and we had this terrible crack of thunder and I woke up and he was dead at that time. His eyes were in the position they should be. Which was a strange thing. Here for two months I had been worried because here was this man with his eyes rolled back up into his head when I'd get up in the morning, and then when he did die, the eyes were open but staring straight ahead. So sometime in that two hours he had died.

The hospice people had told me that once he was dead to make sure he was dead because otherwise when EMS came you would have a problem if they could resuscitate him. I don't know how long he had been dead. I knew he had been alive two hours before—he was still warm. But when they came in they didn't even consider that he could be alive. I had called hospice; I called the lady who had cared for him because she said she would come over, and I called this neighbor and she came. That was fine because I knew them, but somehow the idea of being with a bunch of strangers really bothered me. When the EMS people came they were very nice and supportive.

The undertaker did not come; well, they came just before my daughter had to leave for school. Thank God. I was very glad because she also heard the crack of thunder and when she woke up she knew he was dead. I don't know why, but she did not want to come and see him, and the only way to get out of the house was past the bed.

In terminal illness you have more time to talk about it. I went through this with my father and was in the room when he died. Death is never easy. It was definitely a relief. I don't feel I have had guilt feelings. I understand a lot of people do. The nicest thing that could have happened was for him to die. If I could have him back the way he was, I would love it.

I definitely feel he was afraid to die for a long time, but don't think he was in the end. I think he wanted to die. In the condition he was in, you probably get to that stage. For a person who was as proud as he was, it was just a terrible way to die because he always had been very proud of his athletic abilities. He was a very intelligent man. Here he was, trapped. You are in this shell and can't get out, and that is where he was, so he struck out at everyone else. No, I shouldn't say that, he struck out mainly at me and my daughter. Which again—they say you hurt the people you love the most.

Joyce Smith

LUCINDA KLEIN: I don't remember when she started talking about killing herself. At some point I decided to stop arguing with her about that. I said, "I won't kill you but I won't fight you." So when she did do it, it was a complete shock because she had been talking about it so much that I didn't think that she was going to do it. I thought it had become—well, that she had gone beyond the point where it would lead to action. I thought there was one thing I could have done as far as real invasive action, I could have called a hospital and told them that she was threatening to kill herself and that I was afraid that she would. I imagine that she could have been committed to a psychiatric ward. But the thought of that to me seemed like the worst kind of—like selling her out in the worst way, just like being a traitor. I just couldn't imagine doing that.

I know one person whose lover tried to kill himself. His lover took an overdose and ended up in the hospital for a month, and it was really helpful. But I think Joyce was forty-six and this man was only twenty-eight. She had a whole lifetime of real difficult circumstances which she had overcome, but I think this was the last blow for her. Whenever I would tell her about AZT* she would say, "Yes, but that is a younger person and I am not so young."

When I stopped fighting her about it, it became very much more peaceful at home and we had at least several weeks during which we could talk about how much we loved each other and how much we would miss each other and acknowledge that she was going to be going even though I still didn't want her to. We were both very committed and politically active. She said, "One thing you have to do is lobby for euthanasia so that people can die peacefully."

We didn't plan it together. I really didn't want her to, the thing that happened. She kept talking about it. She said, "This is the only reason I got out of the hospital." She had a very good point, which was that she was starting to have problems with her vision, which sometimes happens with AIDS. What she feared was, "I will be in the hospital, blind. I won't even know who is sticking needles into me and I won't be able to do anything about it because I will be too weak." She was always afraid that I would abandon her at some point.

*Azidothymidine (AZT) was the first medication approved by the government for controlling the onset and symptoms of AIDS. As of 1998, a new class of antiretroviral drugs called protease inhibitors had had a dramatic impact, slowing the course of the disease and reducing symptoms.

The way I see it, she made a real rational decision to kill herself but that she had to get crazy to do it. It was a real struggle. I saw this struggle going on. I said to her one day, "You are trying to go down two paths at the same time, one towards life, one towards death." We would talk some. I was practically the only person she talked to.

I decided I was not going to try and stop her. I realized that I could not have been in the room and watched her or anything like that because I just—even though I knew how much she wanted to die, when I came in and found her dead, I absolutely wanted her to be alive. It was very bad.

The day that she killed herself, she had asked me to go out and get a calzone. When I came back, she had locked the chain locks. I really thought she was just mad at me because she had told me to not go right then. So I opened the door as much as I could and said I am going out for a walk. This went on for two hours, I couldn't get in. By the time I got in, I thought she was dead. I could understand her being angry for a little and then letting me in, but nothing was changing and I couldn't hear anything. I was afraid to call the fire department because I didn't want strangers to find her.

It is true; she hung herself. She hung herself from the bar, actually strangled herself from the bar above the bed. It was terrible. But I know that it was worse for her. That is not an instant thing. It is painful. It is not like when you hang and lose consciousness. It was very prolonged. She did have pills that she could have taken but she couldn't be sure that they would actually kill her. She could have ended up in a coma and been worse off just being kept alive. To have to resort to things like that!

I tried to call friends when I found her. I knew she was dead. She was hanging there and there was blood trickling out of her mouth. I called a bunch of people and no one was home. Then I called my mother and asked her to come, which she did, and which was very nice. Then the police kept saying, "You have to notify a member of the family." By then a couple of friends had come over. So the police were really on me and I decided to call her half-brother. I couldn't call her father yet because I knew I would have to ask him for money to bury her.

I was afraid to call the police because they wouldn't believe me or would give me a hard time. They were fine; they were nice. There was a zillion here; they were there twelve hours. It was very comforting that she was there for quite a while. I kept going into the living room where she was lying. We—being the cops, my friends, my mother—were all sitting in this tiny kitchen smoking up a storm. I would periodically go in. I had taken her down right away but I was supposed to leave it undisturbed. The detectives would say I wasn't supposed to be there, but the regular policewoman was very compassionate; so I would go in and sit with her.

I thought a dead body would be very scary but it wasn't at all. It's much different than you would imagine. It was her, I could feel that she was starting to cool off and I could begin to see some discoloration from the strangulating but I held her and kissed her. I would have found it horrible if she had been gone. That would have been just horrible. I think accidents—if someone dies suddenly in an accident it must be much more difficult than if you have a chance to prepare for it. It was her as much as all the other times when I would sit with her and stroke her hair and touch her. It was very reassuring that she was there.

Dorothy Stead

JOE STEAD: When she was up at the hospital the first time and they were going to put her on life support, I said, "No way." If it gets so that the only way she can live is on machines—we both had agreed years ago never to go on a machine. If I go in there and the only way they can keep me alive is on a support system, I don't want it. I don't want the kids or whoever is here to be agonized with my agony. When my time comes, I want to go. I want to live every day that I can. And I am going to. I am a stubborn old shit.

The nurse told me, "I hate to say it, but she is going to go pretty soon." I said, "I know it." So I called the kids. The kids all live near here and they used to come up and sit here and do what they could for their mother. Around Thursday night the kids stayed here, most of them. They slept on the floor; they slept everyplace. I think there were nine of us. Most all the kids stayed here, my grandchildren and kids. Then on Friday I was just walking around, I didn't know what I was doing. I knew what I was doing but I couldn't do what I wanted to do because I was that tired.

The nurse was here. Every day, she either came over here or she called. If I was away, the aide would be here and she would call to find out how things were. Well then, she was here Friday. She was here late and said, "Joe, why don't I call your daughter and have her stay the night so you can get some sleep?" The kids had kinda disappeared and my daughter came over and stayed. Dorothy couldn't drink; she couldn't eat. I would take one of these little things like a toothbrush and I would get that and water and wipe her mouth out and she tried to squeeze the water out of that.

The nurse was here; she would come and look after her. And my daughter was here and my grandchildren were here. I had help to get out of the house for a few minutes on Saturday. She was real bad; she didn't complain, she never complained for the world. I'd go in and talk to her and she would try to smile. Before the time she really got bad, she said, "Why don't you let me go?" I said, "I can't." Then on Saturday morning, my daughter had been here the night before and the nurse called at seven-thirty [and] wanted to know how things were. I said, "We got through the night all right. The kids are here." She said, "I'll keep in touch with you. If you need me, call me." I didn't have to call her: she kept calling here. She came out about seven at night. She stayed right here. I would come out here and the nurse and one of the kids would be in there, and the nurse came out about ten and said, "I think you had better come in." So all the kids and I went in with the nurse and she helped and we stayed right there with her until she was gone.

There at the last she didn't hurt; she didn't complain. She wasn't in any pain; she didn't take any medicine for pain.

The nurse called the funeral director and then asked if I wanted to stay in here while she prepared her for the funeral director. I said, "No, but if you would do that, I would appreciate it." She cleaned her all up and had her laying in there like she was asleep. The funeral director came in about forty-five minutes. I know him very well; in fact he is a friend of my daughter's. He put her on the gurney and I kissed her good-bye and that was the last I saw of her. That is the only way it could happen. It would take so long to get her into clothes and see that she was clean. I sent the wig and a pair of slippers and a sweater and the clothes the daughter and I felt were appropriate. We took her rings off. I have her glasses. The nurse was right in there until the funeral director drove up. As I said, she was well prepared.

I can still see her lying there and some of the things she did before she passed away. I was holding her in my arms and talking to her when she died. The nurse told me to keep talking to her right until the last minute because they can understand. My children talked to her. They talked to her first and I was right there with her when she passed on, passed away. I told her I was going to stay here and not to worry that everything would be all right. I said a little prayer and after she passed away I got the kids out in the living room and we prayed. I told them what I was going to do so they would know. They respected my wishes. At that time I was bad but I was very calm in my ways, which was hard to do especially looking at all these grandchildren. The youngest one there was twenty.

We have two younger grandchildren but we didn't let them see Grandma. They were over here while she was sick, but she could talk to them and play with them. When they went home I told the daughter-in-law that Grandma was very bad and when she passed away I called right away and told her. And then she explained to the kids that Grandma had gone to heaven. I think that was better because they remember when Grandma would do a little coloring for them or give them some candy or gum for them, sugar-free gum.

David Steiner

BONNIE STEINER: It was great the day he was home. It was a nice day. It had rained during the day, and I took him out and let him play in the grass sitting under the trees. We had some ducks out in the pond and we went out and fed the ducks and he giggled and laughed.

He took a nap that night and I fell asleep on the bed with him. Jack said my legs were hanging off the bed, I was so tired. I fell on the bed and fell asleep and he woke me up to see if David needed something. I ended up getting him up. He started crying and he was just screaming. He had become very constipated and was vomiting and on diuretics. He was straining hard to have a stool and I picked him up and he had a seizure. That scared me; he just started breathing funny and was seizing, so I put him back down and then he kind of breathed out and then started to come around again, and I picked him up again and he died. He took three or four very long gasping breaths—no more seizing—and that was it and that is how he died.

It was very quick and I would rather have had him die the way he did—very quickly in a matter of a minute or two—than to go on and suffer like they said he would, in stages.

About two weeks after this, I read about infant cardiology and realized what had happened. A blood clot had gone to the brain, and that was the brain's reaction in effect because of the position I put him in, but that is how I always picked him up to hold him up here on my shoulder, that was just very natural. But I sat here and cried for hours.

After David died, I had Jack call the nurse and she came running right out. As soon as David died, I came out carrying him and crying and I just stood there and Jack said, "Is he dead?" and I said, "Yes." He ran down in the basement; he is a very squeamish man and there was no way he could deal with it. I had said to call the nurse because I wanted her to be here if she could. So she came out in half an hour or forty-five minutes and she was very good.

I was concerned because I hadn't bathed him. I had been bathing him like every other day in the hospital and I had meant to bathe him the next day. I hadn't bathed him and for some reason that bothered me. I don't know why that bothered me, but it did. I mentioned it to her and she said, "Let's give him a bath right now; we can do that." So she helped me bathe him and said we should cut a little hair off so we could save some hair, because we were going to have him cremated.

Jack would just leave the room whenever he saw him. He liked seeing me hold him but there was no way that he would. He finally came up after about an hour and wanted to look at him for about a minute but that was as close as he could get. Finally the nurse said, "Would it be all right if I held him for a little while?" She said she thought that might give Jack permission to ask, so within a little while he came up and asked if he could hold him and he brought him out here by himself and just sat and talked to him and we left him alone. He held him for quite a while. He held him at the funeral home, too.

The nurse said I could hold him all night if I wanted to; I didn't have to give him up; we would call when I was ready. I finally got tired around 4 A.M. She said, "If I get tired, I will just curl up on the couch—it's fine." She stayed here, and then we called the funeral home and they got here about 4:30. They had this great big empty hearse; they put him in the back and I wrapped him up. If I hadn't been so tired—one of the things I said to the nurse after they left was, "I wish we had taken him there because that really bothered me." She went in to talk to them [afterward] and they purchased a bassinet for picking up babies, because that just really bothered me; that was really hard to put him in the back of the hearse.

I was not anxious about him dying at home. I had seen lots of people die and been in lots of codes and had my mother-in-law die at home. It made me very comfortable to have him die at home.

Herbert Wolf

HELENA WOLF: There were two distinct things I remember. One was a number of years before, we had a friend of ours who was dying of breast cancer, and I went to see her the afternoon before she died. This was excruciating at best, as you can imagine, to see a woman your age with children the same age as yours dying of cancer. When I saw her, her cancer had metastasized to her liver and she was incredibly jaundiced. Her eyes were yellow with red spots. You have never seen someone look like this until you have been to see someone that sick. One day, about ten days before Herbert died, I went into his room and he looked the way my friend had looked. That was the day I knew he wasn't going to live for the next three months, that he had suddenly become dramatically sicker. That was certainly one indication, and that certainly forced me to reevaluate what was happening. And the second was the agitation, which was the impetus for putting him in the hospital.

When my father was dying, especially right at the end when he started to slip into the coma, there was this sort of overwhelming feeling that I had that he was going someplace. You never had this sense that he was going to be dead and it was going to just stop like someone turning off the light. There was this enormous sense that he wasn't going to be there in his body but he was clearly going to go someplace. Certainly, I mean, I am not a religious person, I don't believe very much in heaven, but certainly I had an enormous sense that he felt that as well. We took pictures to the hospital and he would talk about them: "I want to see the pictures; I need to have lots of pictures to take with me." He said that more than once—"Where are all the pictures? I need thousands of pictures." Then he said he was going to have Luigi's pizza, his favorite. He said, "When I get to heaven, I am going to have Luigi's pizza." I think that for him, from what was going on in the inside, it must have been like going to sleep. The body is a wonderful thing; it lets you—at least sometimes—it lets you slip away in a very peaceful way.

Thursday morning he couldn't be roused; he was clearly in the final stages of dying. He did not talk to me. They didn't—I don't remember —I don't think they medicated him. Kurt, my brother, and I stayed at the hospital; we sat with him until about lunchtime, waiting for the doctor to come. We talked to him; we talked about what he thought. He couldn't really tell; [our father] might live an hour or a few days, clearly not longer. Clearly they weren't going to do anything. Before, there had been some discussion of whether they would move him. Clearly those issues were no longer of importance. He wasn't going to go anywhere, and moving him down the hall, let alone to another facility, would have killed him.

Finally, about two, two-thirty, we decided to leave; there wasn't anything to be done for him. We decided to go and get a bite of lunch. Then we bought watches for everyone at a discount store. We were just killing time. We got some lunch. We came home and called the hospital and he had died an hour before. He died about four in the afternoon; he just stopped breathing, which is what we had expected would happen. There was nothing very dramatic about it. We got in the car and went back to the hospital. Philip came with us. He had already made some arrangements with the funeral home to take—to transfer—the body.

I don't have a whole lot of regrets about not being with him at the end sort of stuff. We were with him at the end as far as he was concerned. I think at that point we—it had been, you know, just enough. At least I was so thoroughly worn out emotionally I am not sure I could have sat in the room with him and watched him die. I was comfortable with the fact that he did not know what was going on. I felt that I could go away from that. I never went to see him; both Philip and Kurt went into the room to see him. I couldn't go. And you know, they said he looked peaceful.

I think you just have to go real easy and let the kids deal with it in their own way. We talked to them and we tried to be as open as possible with the kids about what was wrong with him. But because of this issue of trying to protect his privacy, we tried to get them to understand that they shouldn't run to school and tell their friends that their grandfather was dying. Laura perceived that we knew things that we weren't telling them, and of course for a long time we didn't know what was happening. When it became clear that he was going to die, we did tell them, but it was couched as gently as possible—you know: "Grandpa isn't going to get better." Laura was quite angry. "Why isn't he going to get better? Isn't there anything they can do?" Gregg was more philosophical. We didn't push them to be overly involved. They still had their lives. They were still going to school. Only time will tell whether we struck the right balance. It was hard and there is no question that we certainly felt it afterwards.

When it was going on, I went to school and talked to their teachers and told them what was going on at home both when he was sick and after he died because I felt that they should be aware of it.

John Wright

HELEN WRIGHT: We just knew. He really couldn't eat much; nothing would stay down. It just didn't work—the food—nothing worked. He urged the doctor to let him come home. And so the doctor agreed.

He didn't get into the wheelchair immediately, but very soon. He went down very rapidly that last week. We had wonderful drives to see the spring flowers. It was in April. The magnolia was coming into bloom, and the crocus in the neighborhood, and we went to some of the beautiful places in town where the beautiful bulbs are and the flowering trees. Every day we would take a drive. Sunday he went to church and stayed through the service and through a forum on mental illness. Then we took another drive, and he came and took a nap, and then we went to a Community Center board meeting, a group we belong to near here. He had a lot of caring about it and was trying very hard to see we built an addition for a retreat center. He passed on his duties to someone else. Monday he took—each morning he would take [a] walk in the wheelchair and go around the neighborhood. I had broken my arm, so I was in physical therapy every two days, so while the aide was here, I would go to my physical therapy.

He would always sit in here and eat. He would never stay in his room and eat. He would even counsel. I think his last client came on Wednesday afternoon. He was mentally O.K. He even did his income taxes, finished them on Thursday. He sat right there and finished them. I thought later, "How absurd! He shouldn't have been doing that income tax. I could have gotten someone else to do that." But because he had always done it without asking someone else, he wanted to do it. Our son-in-law had helped him in the hospital with the income tax, but he did the final thing. But he enjoyed being very independent, functioning until the very last.

He didn't have the energy by Sunday to say anything. We had had lots of time to talk when he was in the hospital and in the last few years —lots and lots of sharing. So there wasn't a lot of sharing in the last few days; he just didn't have the energy to do anything but just exist.

My youngest son came on Wednesday, the next youngest came Thursday, and my daughter came Friday. The other son and his wife had just had a baby a few days before, but they made it by Sunday morning.

My oldest son is kind of good at having good ideas. He is very creative—and everybody does what they see to do but they don't have new ideas. But he was sure it would be a good idea to have people from church come in and have a service for worship on Sunday afternoon. Even though we all knew that he was very, very ill, you never quite— you never knew when it was going to happen, so you keep projecting life into the future. I said, "I don't think we should have the group come because he said he didn't think he needed any more visitors: We are just going to be home together now." But Lee asked him and he said, "Yes." That was all he could say; that was about the last word he ever said. He couldn't talk anymore; his speech was failing. He would say, "Yes" and "No." So we got in touch with some people. They were just the right people. We had about twenty people here. They came in and sat over here and all around there, and he sat over there. He came in about two and they came about four. We played some Bach, some things that had some special meaning for us, and we had quiet worship and everybody got to say good-bye as they came, because they knew somehow that it was good-bye. We played "The Lark Ascending," and there was ministry and quiet and singing. Lee is great at singing. He and his wife do a lot of singing, know lots of songs. So people left about five-thirty, one by one. We ate supper and he just sat there.

The nurse had come in—we had asked to have a nurse stay overnight, so she had come in. We were all just kind of moving around, we were all kind of exhausted and he was just quiet. We decided that he and I would go to bed, so the boys helped to put him in the wheelchair and took him in. It was very difficult; they had to totally lift him, and as soon as he got in bed, he died.

We were all right there—we all went there immediately. All of us were in the house; we all went there immediately. The nurse said, "He's dying," so we all went there. She just knew that; he just went very fast. I don't know whether we actually—who knows, but we were there. Mostly it was here that we were with him. You know he was conscious. His various senses were failing but he could still hear us. I think the sense of hearing goes last. So he could hear the music and hear what we had said and he continued to use his hands, a kind of talking with his hands. But it seemed like he couldn't see us anymore.

We stayed with him until twelve. The nurse said it was O.K., that we didn't have to call the funeral home. She did all the work of calling the doctor and signing the papers. It was really good to have her here, really wonderful.

I was glad the nurse made it clear there didn't need to be any rush. I spent the last half-hour with him alone before they took his body out. The boys and our daughter took him out. They wrapped his body up in a sheet and carried him out. We had a very wonderful Bach thing going real loud and we flung the door open. My neighbor heard the music and must have been up and saw the funeral director's car come in and saw us go out. Lee picked a daffodil and put it on top of the hearse and

said, "Bye Daddy." It was very celebratory. It seemed really good that
he was dying and that he somehow chose to die before it got worse. It
seemed like he was participating and not just a passive victim.

He was giving his body to be used by the medical school. I had
arranged for him to be taken to the funeral home when he died, and
they would transport the body because we are not allowed to transport
the body. The medical school is not allowed to receive bodies except
through the funeral director. So, fortunately, I had arranged for all that.
I found the cheapest funeral home. I was so delighted. So they came at
twelve and took the body.

I wasn't exhausted afterwards. I was on a kind of high for quite a
while. I had gotten myself into a state, and it took a while to get to the
layers of sadness that had been covered over.

The grandchildren were very fond of John. He had developed a
very close relationship with them, even with the two-year-old. They just
ran in and out. It was spring, so they would play outdoors and they
would come in and bring some flowers for him. They really enjoyed
each other; they were fond of each other and had lots of contact with
each other even though they didn't live real close. They had had time
together. They were aware of it being a serious time but they didn't stay
constantly. John looked really, really bad, very diminished, emaciated.
They were, they just kind of kept on playing around.

The six-year-old girl couldn't understand why we were singing after John died. Lee is a great song leader, so we sang after John died,
from nine on. She drew a picture with all the grown-ups smiling and all
the children crying. She said, "Why were we crying and you were all
smiling?"

Deaths that are not sudden but rather the result of the disease process are a transition. It is difficult to say when any particular person
begins actively to die—that is, when key physical functions cease to
work. Sometimes it is a matter of hours, sometimes days. Often the
dying remain alert enough to communicate with caregivers, although often their attention is focused inward. The analogy to giving birth is quite accurate here. The person must work to die in the
same way that a woman labors to give birth. It is a stressful, invol-
untary, but entirely natural process. In the end, life ceases. But what
is finally and absolutely over is only the farthest extremity of life.
Much of what constitutes life, as well as the identity of the person,
has already ceased to exist. For those who are religious, this process

can involve a growth of a spiritual identity as the person moves from the world of the living into that of the dead. Caring for someone at home allows the caregiver to participate in this transition: as it were, to accompany the dying person to the very end of the journey through life.

CHAPTER SEVEN

After Death

This brief final chapter has three sections. The first, on the funeral, continues the theme of the book: that the dying and their families can take control of the dying process, and in this case can extend that control to the funeral or memorial service. In so doing, they can infuse it with meaning that is unique to the dead person and the individual circumstances. This can also be done within a traditional ritual context and framework.

The second section of this chapter allows the reader to follow the caregivers presented in the book through their grieving. It is a just and appropriate end to the reader's witnessing of these intensely intimate and powerfully significant experiences in the caregivers' lives.

There are of course numerous practical matters that must be dealt with when someone dies. This is the topic of the final section. Many of these, primarily the transfer of assets, can and should be attended to while the person is still alive, preferably while he or she can sign documents.

The Funeral

Funeral directors are increasingly becoming aware of and sensitive to people's desire to retain control over the funeral process, beginning with the removal of the body from the home. It is possible, for instance, to specify that the body be removed from the home with the face showing, like a patient being taken away by ambulance. This greatly diminishes the trauma caused by the use of a body bag, the common way of removing the body. If this would be important to the caregiver and family, it must be specified in advance.

One of the advantages of an anticipated death is that the funeral can be planned. Although it may seem difficult, or as one informant said, "ghoulish," to plan the funeral before the person dies, there are a great many advantages in doing so. For one thing, the caregiver and family, or someone acting on their behalf, can interview different funeral directors to determine who will best meet the needs of the family and fulfill the dying person's wishes. Most important is that the dying person can participate in the planning and can specify what kind of remembrance, if any, should take place, and what should be done with the body. For example, such decisions as whether the body should be viewed and how, and the conduct of the memorial service—what music, whether there should be prayers (and if so, which ones), or readings, who should speak—can be made by the dying person.

Another advantage of planning ahead of death is that it frees the grief-stricken caregiver from having to make decisions and take responsibility for the planning. As I have noted elsewhere, many caregivers in this study were surprised by the intensity of their grief, believing that in their prolonged exposure to the dying process they had somehow already encountered their grief. For most of them, this was clearly not the case, and not having to deal with funeral preparations was a great relief.

LUCILLE DeMOTT: Jim and I had spent a lot of time dealing with the death issue. He wasn't sure what he wanted to have done at his funeral and burial. We had invited a minister to lunch to talk about the issues and options as we went through the process. One of Jim's friends was a minister, too. He would come over and the three of us talked about death and the meaning of life together. Out of these discussions Jim designed his own funeral. One of the marvelous things which happened was that a music group which we had asked to play at his funeral came and played chamber music in his bedroom. We got to thinking that it was no fun for Jim not to be there in the sense of hearing it. So they played a whole lot of music at our home, in his room; he chose what he wanted to have played at his funeral.

The funeral was held in a church, but it was a celebration of life as opposed to the tragedy of death. He had selected people to talk about him that he had known for many years. They were just wonderful talks. They were descriptions of him in a lot of different situations. There was the chamber music too. At the cemetery he wanted New Orleans jazz, so we had a jazz band there playing all the wonderful New Orleans jazz music. There was a lot of sadness, but also it was a joy to be able to be cognizant enough to plan all of this, to get settled whatever religious and life meaning issues we had. It helped me tremendously because we did so much discussion of really important issues. I might add all of this occurred after some doctors had advocated for his death.

The baby went to the funeral with a caretaker, and she went to the cemetery. Philip actually placed the ashes in the ground. He wanted a role in the service and we had spent a lot of time talking with him about it. Jim asked him to place the urn in the ground. When we were planning the service, Philip wasn't sure he could do it, so he had an option. He decided he wanted to do it. He played his part very well. A few months later we went back to the cemetery. It was the first time the kids had visited. Ruthy went through the whole burial service all over again with her teddy bear. She put her teddy on the grave. She had remembered and watched the whole thing and redid it. I think it is important to have kids participate.

LUCINDA KLEIN: This whole thing with her family was so weird. She was in touch with her adoptive father. She knew her natural mother and those children. Her brother was in town but he wouldn't come and visit because he was afraid of AIDS. Her adoptive father is very old. She didn't know where her adoptive mother was. Initially her family wasn't involved in the death. My mother and I went to a funeral home nearby and one which was good in handling AIDS patients. We found out how much it would cost for a funeral. Joyce and I had talked about it a little bit. What she said was, "I'll get cremated because it is cheaper." I said, "Wouldn't you like to have a gravestone?" I said, "Everyone has a gravestone." She will have a gravestone. She doesn't yet, but she will.

I had to do everything. Then I called her father and told him how much money I needed. This other relative, a really horrible man who had abused Joyce when she was little—I had to call him because he was here. I called him and he said, "That amount sounds fine; my father will send it tomorrow." Then late that night her adoptive mother called and said that the family wanted to bring her down to South Carolina to be buried there. I wanted her to be buried here, but they are her parents so I left it at that. We went to the funeral home the next morning. Then the family started in about where she would be buried. At that point I just let them do it, and I held a wake.

I did this thing, I asked people to write something about her and then I collected them. So I have these nice things. This is for me.

MARY ROEHM: The funeral home had a family night, one night when just our family could be there and the kids could ask questions. My grandson wanted to know if Grandpa had his shoes on or trousers on so we showed him. Things like that give them a whole different feeling. The littlest girl wanted to crawl right in with him. The seven-year-old whispered to me, "Do you know what I did? I put my picture in Grandpa's pocket." The undertaker wanted us to bring pictures. My daughter made up a scrapbook and we made a composite of the pictures and put that on the coffin. They all wanted to be there. Tim, our son-in-law, asked if we would put Grandpa's cap on in the casket because he remembered Grandpa with his cap on. So we did that. More people remarked about that—that it looked so right on him. We couldn't feel grateful enough to the funeral directors. That helped us over the bridge.

FLORENCE MARTIN: I had, since I knew he was terminally ill, which he did not know—but I had made a lot of the funeral arrangements beforehand and I am so glad I did. It really helped. Even the couple of decisions which I had to make, that I hadn't made before, I had trouble making, and I don't have trouble making decisions. But I was so worn out and so stressed out and everything else. This way it was all taken care of and I just didn't have to do things.

I had made him decide what he wanted done. He said he wanted to be cremated. I said, "I want this said in front of every single member of your family before you die so that there is no problem afterwards." Because it was a second marriage, I didn't want repercussions coming back: "We didn't want him cremated and you did it." So by doing this ahead of time it was just so much easier. I wasn't—I still was upset doing it, but it wasn't the same idea and I have heard people say it is so much harder to make decisions afterwards.

We had a memorial service; he did not want to be shown, which was fine with me. I definitely agreed with that. We had the service a week later, which was nice; it gave me time to get more rested. Three of his kids were able to come in; the fourth one was not able to come. My neighbors all got together and we had everybody back to the house afterwards. We had a hundred to a hundred and fifty people here. His kids from out of town stayed here. To me it was so much easier—it was hard, but so much easier doing it ahead of time.

BONNIE STEINER: I felt a really great need to hold him. I walked in and saw him in that casket. I had said I wanted a closed casket and they just said, "Well he was just such a pretty baby; and he looked so good." They felt maybe I would change my mind and have the casket open. They said they felt it was really better in the long run to have the casket open. I went along with that, but when I saw the casket open, it was real hard to see him in there. I just felt like I wanted to hold him; so whenever I could I would take him out and hold him. Whenever there was no one there, I would take him out and hold him. I really think that helped me a great deal.

What we did during some of the visitation time was—I had a lot of encouragement to take him out and hold him. So, what they did was—we were in a big enough room so that we would enclose a portion, and then one of my friends—whenever someone came, would close the partition and would go out and say that I was holding David and that if the person felt all right about coming in they were welcome to do that. If not, I would be out in a few minutes and she would tell me who was there. It was great, really helpful.

There was one lady who wanted to come in and see me and she didn't want to make a fuss, but I knew she had a real hard time with it because she just went, "Ah," and I could see she was thinking, "How did I get into this?" But other people had an O.K. time and would just sit there and it seemed so natural to see me holding him. It made it more comfortable for all of them and it also made it very easy.

Other than that, the main complaint I had about the funeral home was the funeral director seemed irritated every time I wanted to pick him up. I think he was afraid there was going to be a release of some bodily fluids. They came out at one time and he said, "I was afraid that was going to happen." He just seemed very irritated with me that I would do it, but he couldn't really come out and say, "Please, we don't pick up the bodies around here," or whatever. But he just seemed very like, "Uh, she's in there holding him again," or something like that. I could just tell by his manner that he wasn't happy with me, but that is what I felt comfortable with. I knew I had better get it all out of my system because there was going to come a time soon when I wasn't going to be able to do that anymore. In fact, I held him during the funeral service. Jack asked me if I would. He said, "Do you mind if just you and I are back here?"—because we had people like my dad and various other people who were going to come back and sit with us in this little area for the family. He said, "Do you mind if it's just you and me and you hold David?" We pulled the curtains and nobody really knew. I sat there and held him through the whole service.

We packed a lot of stuff in the casket—you know, toys and his favorite mobile, and a picture of both of us that we signed, his favorite blanket, and all sorts of things. The hardest thing was walking away at the end of the service and knowing that that was going to be the last time I was going to be able to look at him. For some reason that was real hard; that was good-bye.

For people who lose kids, it is helpful to know that it is O.K. to hold them; that is their child and the funeral home can't tell you not to do that. It helped me immensely to do that. I know one woman who didn't even see her child after he died, and I think she had some lingering problems from that. It must have been helpful in the old days for people to keep their loved ones at home. In fact my girlfriend had said, "You know David is still your child. If you want to take him and keep him at home with you it's O.K. No one can tell you you can't." She had just been through this business when her husband died where they had placed all this makeup on him and she had gone and washed it off. I ended up doing that with David because they had makeup on him.

PAT KNOTT: We had Lisa cremated, which was difficult for some people, but it was something we had discussed along the way and was something we wanted to do. We have her remains buried in a little country cemetery near here where my mother is buried and my father will be buried. It's a lovely little spot, very "countryside." We had a service for my extended family at the grave side—a little grave-side service just for family.

We had a memorial service at our church. I didn't want to go through with that, and I can remember my father saying, "It will be good for you to go through with this," and saying to him, "I don't want to go." It was Tuesday and she died on Saturday and I just thought, "I can't face any more people; I don't want to talk about this again." But I think it is a good thing to do; and in fact sometimes I notice in obituaries that people don't have any services and I wonder. I think there is a certain amount of resolving or accepting things which takes place in a funeral. When you go through with those kinds of services, it is not a comfortable thing to go through but it helps.

Grief

This section recounts the grieving of some of the informants in the book. It is not intended to be a systematic discussion of grief. It is, rather, a logical conclusion to the process of caring for a dying person. These people were interviewed at points ranging from six months to five years after the death of the person they cared for. Their stories represent different experiences with grieving and stages of grieving. This material is presented to demonstrate the range of experience and to document the intensity of grief even years after a person has died.

With the exception of Helen Wright, all the informants felt that American society in general is unsympathetic to those who are grieving. There was a uniform assessment that outsiders expected someone to grieve for three weeks after the death and then to get beyond it. Recent research has shown that intense grieving lasts from three months to a year and that many people are seriously grieving for two years. Because of the lack of public affirmation of this extended process, these people sometimes felt there was something wrong with them because they were intensely grieving for such a long time after the death. These brief accounts are designed to show that most people do grieve intensely and for an extended period. In traditional societies formal bereavement lasts at least one year. With increased understanding about the dynamics and intensity of grief, perhaps American society will become more sympathetic to people at such an extremely difficult time in their lives.

STAN CLARK: It was all new. We had no parents or anyone who had died, just dogs, and I was really upset for days when the dogs died. I really had no experience with death and dying. We had no religious affiliation of any kind so we had none of that belief system or superstition—whatever you want to call it. We had just operated on the premise that we were immortal and that the whole world was there for us. She was a professor and I an attorney. We sort of had all this wonderful stuff that we did that was so important, and we felt we were so clever.

I think that after she died my compulsion was to continue to see people all the time. If I didn't keep on seeing people, I might fall into this thing of the isolated widower who gets cut off from all previous relationships that he had when he was married. So I think I probably was denying a whole lot of my grief by staying busy and seeing people.

I had three automobile accidents that year because I was distracted and not thinking about things like driving. They weren't serious but indicated my lack of concentration. When I finally started feeling better, I realized there was a whole other mental track going on with me all the time in my head. I was surprised at how bad I continued to feel when she died. I had thought I was in physically, mentally, and emotionally good shape. I was a competent person and I was in good shape. I had no feelings of regret that something had been neglected or that we hadn't had time to say anything we wanted to say—all that stuff. But it was three years before I was really O.K. Later I realized I was scared in general; I had a real paranoid affect. I really missed her, missed talking to her. I [had just become] aware of these uncertain and lonely feelings when they became less constant in my head.

When she got sick, my marriage and what I had with her was the most important part of my life. But it hadn't always been that way. My job, and working, had always been ahead of that. I—we always enjoyed politics and talking about social concerns and political actions we supported, but our personal talking and fine-tuning was at a higher peak by then. In our times at home together we had our routines, which really meant a lot to me. The absence of that everyday talking and those routines was why I was in so much trouble that I didn't realize I would be in after she died. I hadn't recognized their importance to my sense of well-being.

I saw myself as an independent person who had lived alone and already knew he could handle it. I didn't want to lose her but I thought I would be O.K. about it. But it was much, much more devastating than I had imagined, the loss of her being there for me. I think it was because I didn't realize how dependent I was on all this nurturing as a source of my own energy and purpose. She was producing almost at the same rate I was [the] conditions that supported me, little things that someone notices like "You got that in" or "That is interesting after all the trouble that he has given you about that." All those little feedback things or recognitions that have to do with everything that you have known together.

The friends who had been involved in her care helped. All these people said how they had been affected by Alice's and my relationship and our marriage. People talked a lot about that how good it was to be around us. That awareness of your own mortality makes it possible for you to be less petty and more basically concerned about what is a good thing to do and what doesn't matter.

LAURA SWEET: I had no concept of grief at all. I hadn't had anyone in my family or anyone close to me die at all. I had only gone to one funeral in my life and it was someone I didn't know and I was more curious to see the corpse than anything else. The real shock came after he died. It is still a shock to feel these feelings. I always thought, like everyone else in the society who has never experienced death, that you are sad at the funeral and then in three to four weeks you are back to normal; but that is not just the way it goes.

I decided to go to this new job. I had been wanting to go back to school and had put it off for two years to care for Tony. I like to write articles and fiction and was looking forward to being free of that burden. I love Tony, you know, and he wanted me to have a better life. He wrote me a beautiful letter which said he wanted me to have a better and happier life and wanted me to be successful. He didn't want me to have to go on doing this, and he knew that it was really hard on me and appreciated what I did for him.

After Tony died, I was scared; I was afraid of the dark again. I was afraid I was going to see him again. He told me he would come back. I said, "If you can come back, come back and see me but don't scare me." He would scare me after we saw scary movies. I was always scared, and I was scared he was going to play a practical joke after he died and come back and scare me and do this little thing with his finger like they did in *The Shining*. I said, "Don't come back and scare me," and he said he would never do that. "If you can come back, do, because I want to know if you are O.K." So far he only came back to me in a dream. It was really intense and vivid and I felt the next day that he was O.K. It was really a communication of some kind.

Having all my stuff packed up and living with my sister is good. I couldn't have lived in our apartment after he died. I still have to face the hurdle of having to live with our things. Things will remind you at first but after a while they will stop. It is just the first time when you come across them. I have never lived alone. I would have been very, very scared if I would have been with Tony alone in the apartment when he died. Even the night he died, I couldn't sleep in that room. I went in the next night and I couldn't sleep in that room, and I couldn't even go in that room for a while, but now I can.

HELENA WOLF: Afterwards I was just numb—very numb—for a long time. I think I was more emotionally and physically involved in something that was happening to someone else than I had ever been before in my whole life, maybe than I ever will be again, but I don't know about that.

What was the most remarkable thing was how overwhelming it was: both how overwhelming it was while it was going on, then how it consumed you when it was over. I always thought of myself as a competent, logical, rational relatively well-integrated person, and I guess we all have ideas of who we are, based on the situations we have been exposed to up until that moment, and nobody can ever prepare you for the confrontation with loss and the grief that comes with it. You can read about and fantasize what it would be like, but it is too terrible to experience so you don't. You try to make analogies like what it was like when you went to college. But what you can't imagine is the punch line, that you may be away but there is always a letter, a phone call; there's always going to be a response to something you do because the person is still there.

I think the most overwhelming feeling is the sense that something would happen and there wouldn't be anyone there to respond. It wasn't the sense that you needed that person so much to do things for you in your life, but that there is this void, that you talk and no one would answer. That forced a kind of self-reliance that I certainly had never had to experience in my life. If the person you cared for and lost was very close to you, you don't transfer those feelings to someone else, you don't say, "Now I'll have this relationship with someone else," because what you have to confront is the end of that relationship.

It was an overwhelming feeling of my own mortality because, when you have that linkage to someone else, you have that sense of immortality and a sense that you carry the vestiges of that person within you and so that if something happened to you, it is as if two people were being lost. That was a very scary feeling. I'd never had those sensations before. It forced me to think very hard about myself and about integrating what I cared for about my father into my own life, making sure that those things were not only integrated into my own life but were carried on, remembered and reflected by others, not only people that he knew but people that he didn't know. I mean things like: I talk about my father all the time because he was important; he was enormously important to me. He was a very wise person.

It's funny—I always think of a story that my boss once told about her grandmother, who lived well into her nineties and died not long ago. One day she was someplace and told the story that her grandmother had died and the person she told the story to said, "Well, how old was she?" and she said, "Ninety-seven." The person said, "Well, that's all right. She lived a good life." My boss said, "No, every day that she is not alive, I miss her. If she lived to be two hundred and died, I would still miss her." I think that we make the assumption that that was good enough—you have lived long and we can accept those things. But in fact it isn't always true and you don't want people to go away.

It is also, I think, the sort of cliché things which can make you take stock because you realize they are very true. You don't realize how true the clichés are until you have to think about them. I make a very conscious effort to keep up with some of my father's close friends because I care and because that is a link one does not often get. I think you have an appreciation for a wider view, that you must reach out, that you must have a community of people you care about, that you are in touch with, that you share things with. Because if you are able to open up enough about yourself, you have no choice but to expose your own hurt and sorrow. That's a very humbling experience and cuts the wheat from the chaff among your friends: who is willing to watch and who finds it just too painful and just goes away, and who didn't want to see, and those who sort of stuck it out and said, "We understand just how painful this can be."

BONNIE STEINER: I kept feeling that, well, I can rest when this is over, I can cry when this is over. He's gotta see his old mom here and I can't be hanging over him crying all the time. Once he just looked at me when I was crying, right after we had gotten the diagnosis, and he just looked at me so strange, like he had never seen me like that. I just decided then that I really couldn't deal with grieving at that point; I just had to try to not do any of that around him. I didn't want to add any more stress to what he was feeling.

Jack and I were really suicidal for about five to six weeks. We talked about suicide every single day; that is how we got through it. One of us would say, "I can't stand feeling like this. I just can't stand it." The other would be up enough to say, "Let's see how we do; let's get through the afternoon and if we can't stand it tonight we can always do something then." That is how we got through five to six weeks. A lot of this was our not going day to day but thinking, "How will I live the rest of my life without this child?" It was very, very difficult to think in those terms.

Jack had a real hard time. He had been laid off from work and given three months severance pay and was just starting with a new company right when David died. They told him he could have two weeks off. He started a new job with people asking, "Oh, are you married, any children?" and having to fill out W-2 forms without exemptions. So he had a terrible time. He would come home and I would be crying and he would say, "What is the matter?" and I would start to tell him, and he would say, "I can't deal with this." He would leave the room; he was afraid if he ever got back down, he would never be able to function at work. There was a lot of trouble of getting our grieving in sync.

PAT KNOTT: After she died, the hardest thing was finding time for ourselves. All these people who had helped—I don't know where they had got the energy because they had their own families and jobs—but they called us and asked, "Why don't you come over for dinner?" or "Let's go to a movie." So we went out and bought bicycles and we've become distance bicyclists. It was our way of gracefully saying, "It's a nice day; we are going to take a bicycle ride this afternoon." It was nicer somehow than saying, "We just want to be left alone" after they had given so much.

It took me a long time, maybe three years, before I could see her healthy, picture her running across the backyard, going for a walk. I would wake up at night and see her in that hospital bed and could never see her any other way. Eventually it happened, but it took a very long time.

I didn't do anything with her room for a while. It just stayed the way it was. The thing I had the hardest time with was her shoes. I had the hardest time with shoes more than anything else. Anytime I would try to do something with her shoes—and I had all the little sizes when I finally got to the point of organizing clothing and putting things away. Somehow her shoes had been active and running and walking and they just meant "alive." I had the hardest time with those shoes. I left her room with the toys—I think it must have been for three or four months. We have these tapes of her talking and we have never been able to listen to these tapes. We know we just can't do it; we just can't quite sit down and listen. We have them, but—

In those days after she died I was very tired and Don was very tired and we took a lot of naps. I remember lying on the couch, and the thing that would wake me up time after time was, I would think Lisa was walking. There was a stair around the corner—that you came down the stairs and down the hallway and into the living room, and I would have this recurrent dream that she was just walking into the living room. It would always wake me up from my nap. I had an experience once; I think there was a real fine line between insanity and sanity at that time. I remember, after she died, walking down past the toy store and I saw a little doll in their window and thought, "I ought to go in and get that for Lisa; she would love it." I was opening the door to the store before it dawned that there was no Lisa to take that little doll home to. It was times like that that you wonder how close you are to being insane.

You are very fragile. Our culture doesn't allow you to really grieve. Some things aren't socially acceptable like screaming and yelling. We are supposed to be controlled; we are supposed to be a self-sufficient, controlled people. You get those things—those things are more ingrained than you wish at those times. I used to say I had a public persona and a private one. Whenever I went out in public, I would try to be as much in control as possible and then I'd go home and fall apart. What you are doing is meeting other people's expectations. What you are doing is trying to be what everyone thought you should be. But there would be days when someone might reach out and say, "How are you doing?" [and] give you a little squeeze on the arm and that would be it for the day. You would be just a pile of tears. I could stay in control as long as some little thing like that did not happen. But that would be just the end when I lost control.

For months after she died, my arms would ache so much to hold her that I got these really strong cramps in them and had to rub them to get them to stop hurting.

Practical Concerns

Before Death

Many of the practical matters listed here can be attended to after the person dies, but there are many advantages to settling these matters beforehand. Most important is for the dying person to participate in the decision-making process. Death is obviously a touchy and difficult thing to discuss, if there is not already open discussion of dying. If the caregiver feels uncomfortable bringing up the subject, the physician or hospice nurse can help facilitate the discussion.

If the person has written a will, many of these decisions have already been made. Drawing up a will is a very good idea for everyone, even people without much disposable property. With the simple computer programs available today, people can draw up their own will. Even if a will exists, however, it may have to be probated, and during this time the survivors may have difficulty getting access to assets and income.

Property can be transferred by removing the dying person's name from assets held jointly, by adding another person's name to assets that the dying person holds singly, or by having the dying person transfer ownership of certain assets, such as a car. Often a lawyer will make a home visit to draw up these documents when someone is dying. If this is not possible, a notary public can come to the home (or hospital room) and help the patient assign a power of attorney to someone else, who can then carry out legal functions for the dying person.

Here are a few steps that can be taken in advance:

- Make sure all joint assets accurately reflect who owns what. Have all appropriate names recorded.
- Register any changes in a deed with the registrar of deeds in the county where the property is located.
- Remove the dying person's name from any jointly held stocks or bonds. Add the names of other appropriate people, such as children.
- Remove the dying person's name from joint bank accounts. Inform the bank of what is happening.
- Check the patient's health insurance to see if the survivors are covered. If not, obtain health insurance for the survivors.
- Transfer the title of the dying person's automobile and house.
- Ask the dying person where any other assets might be located.

After Death

As I have mentioned, any of the steps outlined here can be taken after the person dies, though it is simpler, more efficient, and generally beneficial for the dying person if they are taken while the person is alive. There may also be a tax advantage to transferring assets before death occurs. If the assets were not transferred prior to death and are not jointly held, the survivors will have to wait until the will or estate goes through probate.

To accomplish the various tasks involved in transferring assets and gaining access to survivor's benefits, it will be necessary to have a copy of the death certificate. In some cases, but not all, the copy will have to be certified. Check to see whether the particular office or agency will accept an uncertified copy, because certified ones are costly.

Many people and institutions will have to be notified of the death. Some of these may offer survivor's or death benefits. The following are places that should be notified, if relevant:

- The person's employer. Check here for insurance, death benefits, profit sharing, and pension benefits.
- Social Security. If the deceased was receiving checks, they will have to be stopped. Any checks received after the death must be returned. Ask whether the surviving spouse or dependent children are eligible for benefits.
- Insurance and credit card companies. If the death was accidental, there may be insurance benefits. Check insurance policies to see if there are unused premiums to be claimed. There may be additional benefits from car insurance or the accident insurance attached to some credit card purchases.
- Union, credit union, and fraternal organizations. If the deceased was a member, find out whether there are death benefits.
- Veterans Administration. The survivors of a veteran may be entitled to benefits.

Settling Financial Matters

Collect all money and debts owed to the deceased. Keep a detailed account of all bills, expenses, and income during this period. The cost of caring for the person and the funeral costs may be deducted from the estate when it goes through probate. This is also true of all bills and debts. Pay these as soon as possible and keep a record of all transactions. In paying bills, first check to see if the debt is covered by life insurance. Such debts as mortgages, credit cards, and student loans often are.

If survivors are left without funds as a result of the death, they can apply for emergency funds to the Department of Social Services in the municipality in which they live.

Family members should check to see if they need to change their own wills or the beneficiaries on their insurance policies.

If problems are encountered in any of these areas, seek the services of an attorney.

Documents Needed

When conducting business having to do with survivors' benefits, debt payments, and so on, call the office or agency before visiting, to find out which documents will be needed. If it is necessary to leave a document at the office, *get a receipt*. The following documents or information may be required*:

death certificates (certified, or copies of the original)
Social Security numbers (survivors' and deceased's)
marriage certificate
birth certificate of each child
armed services discharge papers
insurance policies
deeds and titles to property
stock certificates
bank books
wills
recent income tax forms and W-2 forms
Veterans Administration claim number
automobile registration
loan and installment payment books and contracts

Death represents a profound reorganization of the lives of those involved, beginning with the terminal diagnosis and continuing long after the death has occurred. Successfully integrating the death into ongoing life is a task and challenge for all participants.

* This section was prepared with the assistance of Individualized Home Nursing Care, Inc., Ann Arbor, Michigan, July 1986.

Conclusion: Living while Dying

Home death is about living, living while dying. It is a task not easily undertaken but possible to accomplish. It is something people need to consider carefully. Home death is a powerfully significant experience despite the strain, exhaustion, and conflict that sometimes accompany it. Its power lies in the fact that, in the face of certain death, the caregiver can give the person life, that is, the continuation of life as a social being. The dying person can live a social existence until death closes off all forms of interaction.

As death approaches, those attributes that served to define the person to others and to him- or herself gradually diminish or cease altogether. Movement, wit, personality, the mind, the body—all change, and much is lost. Tending a terminally ill patient at home allows the caregiver to help preserve as much of the dying person's distinctive identity as possible. Being in the home keeps the dying person involved in a web of social interactions and relationships long after he or she is actively able to sustain these ties. To paraphrase Helena Wolf: as long as the caregiver interacts with the dying person, he or she is still alive. In most cases, it was this chance to live to the very end of life that the terminally ill sought in home death and that the caregivers were able to provide.

A key aspect of sustaining life was preserving the ability of the dying to make decisions or, when this was impossible, making decisions that were true to their wishes. Autonomy is a crucial cultural value associated with decision making and the ability to control one's life. These are core attributes of an adult identity in our culture and ones that we seek to introduce to children as early as possible. Respecting the person's autonomy, even marginally, serves to maintain him or her as a cultural or human being, as someone still among the living. In contrast, the relative loss of autonomy in an institutional setting such as the hospital or nursing home is a premature social death. One of the things hospitalized terminally ill patients and their families complain of the most is that the staff and sometimes visitors treat the dying as if they were already dead.

Because the experience of a home death is so powerful, it creates stresses and tensions for the people who participate. It is not that these problems should prevent someone from dying at home, although they may; but they should be carefully evaluated. As this book has emphasized in a number of different ways and contexts, home death requires considerable responsibility, effort, determination, and, perhaps most crucially, social support. Helping someone die at home is not something to be undertaken alone by just the caregiver and the dying person. Just as home death represents a tenacious assertion of the dying person's social and cultural identity over the physical reality of terminal illness, so too is the experience a social one for the caregiver. It is significant not only for the material aspect of the support required (which, to be sure, is of very real importance), but also for the sense of community represented by the support, which helps emotionally to sustain the caregiver.

This is not to say that support is easy to obtain or unambiguously positive when it is present. In some cases, usually from those most intimately connected to the dying person, the support can be as fraught with tension as the care itself. Death is the ultimate drama in life. As such, it exposes the friction and antipathy as well as love that imbues any long-term relationship. At a time when caregivers need support the most, sometimes those providing it can disrupt or impede the process of caring for the dying person. Strife is an integral part of life, and the social and emotional disruption at such a vulnerable time is part of the pulling apart and reconstituting of relationships which accompanies death. However, what happens between the caregiver and supporters at this time will profoundly affect the caregiver's adjustment after the death occurs. Those who are surrounded and supported by others will have an easier time adjusting to bereavement than those without support or those in a stressful situation.

Home death is a social experience. It is an attempt to sustain the dying person's social—that is, human—existence until physical death brings that existence to an end. It expresses a sense of community and belonging which physically, materially, and emotionally sustains the caregiver. The technical expertise provided by professionals helps to make this possible.

Home death is also a spiritual experience, in that it is the transition between life and death and, some believe, the transformation into a new form of existence. In this context the social is profoundly linked to the spiritual. The social aspect represents an individual's existence beyond the mere physical, as well as the group's existence beyond that of the individual members.

Home death is one of the most profoundly meaningful experiences in modern society. Tending the dying is an elemental human experience. It links those involved to basic human values and, in so doing, allows them to transcend the sorrow and tragedy of death.

Tasks and Problems of Caregiving

There are many ways to learn techniques of caregiving. If the dying person is going home from the hospital, the nursing staff there can teach the caregiver to perform the more common procedures such as helping the person in and out of bed or a chair, giving shots, inserting a catheter, suctioning, and taking care of a catheter or nasogastric tube. In addition to the formal instruction the nurses provide, watching the nurses tending the patient is an excellent way to learn caregiving techniques. These may also be learned from a home care or hospice nurse or physical therapist in the home, where training is adapted to the caregiver's abilities, the patient's particular needs, and the resources and physical setup of the home. Training in caregiving can also be obtained from the local Red Cross or from the local community college. In addition, the Red Cross and the state department of public health produce training manuals on home nursing.

This appendix is not intended to serve as a definitive description of home nursing, nor is it intended to take the place of formal training in caregiving techniques. Rather, it is provided to serve as a quick reference for the caregiver to use in problem solving and as a reminder of techniques and information learned in a more formal setting.

This appendix was written with the assistance of Frances Cornelius, M.S.N. Information from the following sources was also helpful: D. Coons, L. J. Metzelaar, A. Robinson, and B. Spencer, *A Better Life: Helping Family Members, Volunteers, and Staff Improve the Quality of Life of Nursing Home Residents Suffering from Alzheimer's Disease and Related Disorders* (Columbus, Ohio: Source for Nursing Home Literature, 1986); and American Cancer Society, "Caring for the Person with Cancer at Home."

General Care

Appearance

It is important to encourage the dying person to maintain his or her appearance. Personal grooming rituals such as a morning shave or applying fingernail polish should be maintained as long as possible. At the very least, getting out of bed to dress or change clothes provides a minimal amount of physical stimulation. But maintaining lifelong rituals of dress and presentation of self will also enhance the person's sense of control. The dying may be very sensitive to how drastically their looks have changed. If this is the case, special care should be taken to prevent the dying person from glancing or gazing into a mirror.

When the patient is extremely debilitated and fragile and possibly cognitively impaired, a gown, shirt, or dress slit up the back may ease caregiving routines such as turning or washing, especially if the person is incontinent. This hospital-gown type of clothing allows the patient to preserve some dignity and makes cleaning and changing easier.

Hair should be brushed or combed daily. Brushing stimulates the scalp and helps remove dirt and dandruff from the hair. If the person is mobile, hair can be washed in the sink or shower. When the person is bedridden, a dry shampoo can be used, or a special hair-washing board can be purchased to facilitate shampooing in bed. Some beauticians and barbers will come out to the home to cut hair.

Fingernails that are too long are difficult to keep clean and can scratch. Long toenails and callouses on the feet cause discomfort and make it difficult for the person to walk. Before attempting to remove callouses and cut toenails, soften them by wrapping the feet in warm, wet towels and covering the towels in plastic for fifteen to thirty minutes. The feet can then be rubbed vigorously with a dry towel, and the dead skin will come off. Apply lotion to the feet after they are dry; this will keep them soft. It is much easier to cut the toenails after they have been soaked like this. Trim nails straight across to prevent accidentally injuring the toe.

Hygiene

Keeping patients clean will help maintain their dignity and sense of control over their life. In addition, the daily ritual of bathing will organize the day and provide a diverting activity. Some of the patients in this book were able to walk and thus to take showers or tub baths until a few days before they died. Others needed to be bathed in bed. For those who use the shower or bath, the addition of non-skid mats and a grab bar will help prevent falls. A shower or bath chair, which can be purchased or rented from a medical supply company, can also help prevent falls and, in addition, overtiredness from the bathing process.

When bathing in bed is necessary, special care should be taken to keep the face, armpits, and genital area clean. A hospice nurse can show the caregiver how to wash a person in bed.

A dying person can develop bad odors for many reasons, such as incontinence, diarrhea, intestinal blockage, problems with digestion, poor oral hygiene, and open wounds. For everyone's well-being, the body should be kept clean and the room well ventilated. It is particularly important to clean the patient after an episode of incontinence to prevent damage to the skin. It is also vital to keep the person clean, because the dying person who smells bad tends to become isolated, and this is very detrimental to the individual's well-being. Products are available which bond with odor molecules and neutralize them completely. These can be purchased from a durable medical equipment (DME) company. Rather than disguising the odor with a scent, they eliminate it.

Skin Care

Preventing breakdown of the skin is one of the major concerns of the caregiver. Breakdown can occur very quickly while a person is bedridden, especially when nutritional problems are present. (Nutrition is dealt with in the next section.) The result of skin breakdown is an extremely painful **decubitus ulcer** or bedsore, which is very difficult to heal or keep from enlarging.

To prevent skin breakdown, encourage the person to get up and move around to maintain good circulation; with poor circulation, cells in the skin will die, resulting in the formation of ulcers. When walking is difficult, sitting the patient on the edge of the bed with legs dangling over the side several times a day will provide some relief for the skin. Wheelchair-bound people can raise themselves up by pressing down on the arms of the chair every twenty minutes or so. Those who are too weak to be out of bed or to sit on the edge of the bed must be turned every three hours. Alternate the patient's position from one side, to back, to the other side. Most people prefer to be on their backs, but they cannot be there all the time. When a person is completely bedridden, doing range-of-motion exercises, which move the joints, will enhance circulation and help prevent skin breakdown. Range-of-motion exercises are appropriate for all levels of function and can be taught by a nurse or physical therapist.

Check for red spots where the skin touches the bone: elbows, knees, heels, head, even the ears. Red spots in these areas indicate risk of skin breakdown. As a preventive measure, massage the whole body, including the areas just mentioned, and place padding around the area to remove pressure. Special mattresses (such as an **egg crate mattress,** inflated mattress, or alternating pressure mattress), a water bed, or a sheepskin mattress pad also can help prevent skin breakdown.

Care should be taken when arranging the person that skin does not touch skin: a pillow must be placed between the legs, a folded towel between the arm and body, and the fingers spread out so that they do not touch each other. If a bedsore does occur, the area should be exposed to the air. New types of bandages allow air in while protecting the area. Special pillows for treating bedsores can be used in addition to gently massaging the area around the sore. A hospice or home health care nurse can provide this care or can teach the caregiver how to do it. The **enterostomal therapist** of a DME company is trained in wound care, as are nurses, and can provide consultation in the care of a bedsore. Depending on the company and the nature of the wound, the consultation will be provided at home or in the company's offices. There are many new products for caring for bedsores. Depending on the amount of drainage, some bandages can be left on for days.

Keeping the patient turned frequently is essential in the prevention or treatment of decubitus ulcers. A nurse or physical therapist can teach the caregiver how to do this. Two people should generally do the turning, one on each side of the bed, although one person who is skilled can turn a patient alone. One should normally turn the patient from one side to the back, then next time from the back to the other side. Figures 2 and 3 illustrate the technique of making this half turn. A full turn—that is, from one side to the other side—is required when there is a decubitus ulcer on the back. This is a more difficult turn to perform. The instructions for the half turn can be adapted to

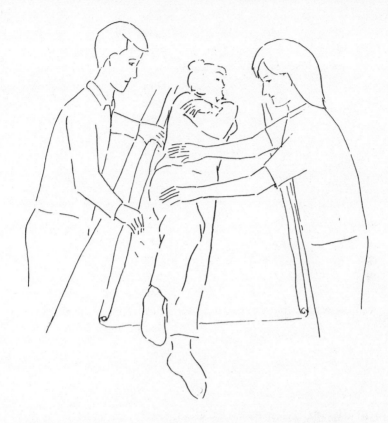

Figure 2. Turning Someone from Her Back to Her Left Side (Step 5)

doing a full turn. Note that in the full turn the person is moved from one side of the *bed* to the other, whereas, in the half turn, the person is moved from one side of the bed to the middle, then, next time, to the other side of the bed.

The steps in making the half turn, as illustrated in figures 2 and 3, are listed below:

1. Move equipment away from the bed. Empty catheter bag (if appropriate) and place it on the side of the bed the person is being turned *to*.
2. Loosen the draw sheet on each side of the person and, on the side *opposite* the one she is being turned to, roll it up to within about ten inches from the body.

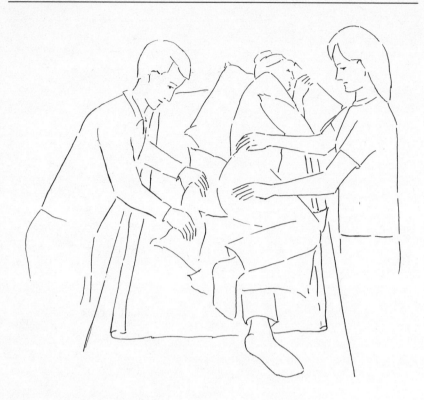

Figure 3. Finishing a Half Turn (Step 6)

3. Cross the person's arms across her body to prevent injury.
4. If you need to move the patient toward the side of the bed *to which she is going*, do so by pulling the draw sheet.
5. Lifting the draw sheet to support her back, roll the person onto her side. This must be done by both attendants *in unison* to keep the patient's back straight (figure 2).
6. Place pillows behind the back to keep the person in place. If necessary, also place pillows between the legs and between the arms and chest to protect the skin (figure 3).
7. Straighten the covers.

If the person has slid down in the bed, one caregiver can reposition her with the help of gravity by raising the foot of the bed and lowering the head. When the move is completed, return the bed to its previous position.

Dying people can be very sensitive to the weight and warmth of blankets. Fold several light cotton blankets at the foot of the bed ready to be put on and taken off as the person's needs change.

The following checklist summarizes for caregivers the essentials of skin care for the terminally ill:

Causes of skin problems:
poor nutrition
lack of exercise
pressure from extended bed rest
urinary or fecal incontinence

Prevention of skin problems:
- Encourage exercise (a bedridden person may sit on the edge of the bed several times a day; if this is not possible, the patient must be turned every three hours).
- Prevent skin from touching skin while the person is in bed.
- Make sure that the bedlinen is straight and that there are no crumbs or wrinkles.
- Use a special padding, such as an egg crate mattress, or inflated mattress pad.
- Watch for redness, especially over any bony prominence. Gently massage areas where redness occurs. Do *not* use alcohol-based lotions because they dry the skin.

Treatment of bedsores:
- Leave the ulcerated area exposed to the air.
- Use special pillows to keep pressure off the area.
- Consult a home care or hospice nurse.

Sexuality

One-third of the couples in this study continued to have sexual intercourse until a few weeks (and, in one case, one week) before the patient's death. The end of the person's desire to have sex marked a clear downturn in his or her condition. The need for couples to continue their sexual relationship should be respected by other family members and caregivers. The couple will need quiet, uninterrupted time. Respecting these needs is part of sustaining the dignity and autonomy of the dying person.

The need for sexual intimacy is most difficult to accept when the individuals are involved in a stigmatized sexual relationship, such as that of a same-sex couple. If caregivers find this objectionable, they need to consider their commitment to the dying person's well-being and decide whether they will be able to respect the person's autonomy and ability to make decisions.

A fatal illness may cause sexual dysfunction. When this occurs it does not mean sexuality ceases. Touching and sensual caressing can have a positive effect on the dying person's well-being and can be an important part of the relationship with the caregiver. Touching and maintaining body contact with the dying person is extremely important.

Health Care

Nutrition

Next to pain control, providing nourishment for the dying person is potentially one of the most frustrating and upsetting caregiving tasks. Not all dying people experience problems in eating and drinking. Some eat normal foods although in drastically reduced amounts, and some maintain normal eating habits until a day or two before death. Most dying people, however, have serious problems eating and drinking. The disease, the treatment for the disease, the medication for pain, and the process of the body shutting down before death can all interfere with eating.

Providing good nourishment is a central aspect of caring for another person. Nourishment is essential to life and often is used to symbolize life itself. In some families nourishment represents the love family members have for one another—a parent's preparation of a meal is a gift of love to a child, and vice versa. When a family member can no longer eat, the concept of the family unit is threatened symbolically, just as it is threatened in reality by the impending death. The caregiver's inability to nourish the dying person may be profoundly upsetting.

Informants undertook to tend the dying in the home to demonstrate their love, but the great difficulty they often encountered in nourishing the patients sometimes frustrated this goal. The frustration was increased, of course, by the very accurate perception that without food and liquid the person would soon die. Nevertheless, *the dying person should never be forced to eat.*

> JOE STEAD: Every day I would try to feed her. And she got so she couldn't eat. She would like to have something and she would start to eat it and she couldn't. I'd fix food that I knew she liked, and she couldn't eat it and I got so down; so far down because I knew that she had to eat. I tried everything.

Causes of an Inability to Eat or Drink
In the dying process the various bodily functions gradually cease. This is known as active dying. As the energy to sustain life diminishes, the body directs what energy remains to maintaining vital functions. Thus the body stops digesting and metabolizing food before the senses stop working or breathing ceases. This process is often complicated by pathological processes associated with the disease or by side effects of treatment such as chemotherapy, pain medication, and radiation therapy.

When the liver is affected as a result of the disease process, the individual's sense of taste can be drastically affected, so almost nothing tastes good. This also can be a side effect of chemo- and radiation therapy. Eating becomes an effort and can cause the person to gag. The same effect can also be produced by an acute sensitivity to smells, which sometimes accompanies disease and chemotherapy.

Nausea is a symptom that frequently accompanies cancer. It can result from the cancer itself, from intestinal blockage, or from treatments such as chemotherapy and radiation. The vomiting that accompanies the nausea can be a serious problem in that it causes the body to lose vital fluids and also makes it impossible for the body to absorb needed medications. In this case other resources of drug administration may be used.

> STAN CLARK: Up until two days before she died, she was eating on occasion an egg, some melon, and a steak. But she was also throwing up and I measured out the stomach contents a lot. I did it because of a concern about loss of fluids and concern about the meds getting down.

Some kinds of chemotherapy, the disease process itself, or infections can cause ulcerations of the mucous membranes in the body. When the individual's body is already in a weakened state, this ulceration becomes more severe. The mouth sores that result are extremely painful and can make it impossible for an individual to eat or take medication orally.

> ANNA KROLICK: My mother would say, "I have to eat; get me something to eat." Then we would try to think of something she would like and would take real care preparing it and carefully disguising the taste of the protein supplement. And she couldn't eat it. She would try but the tears would just run down her face, the pain was so great.

The problem of open ulcers in the mouth must be evaluated and treated on two levels: first, topical anesthetics are needed to allow the person to eat; second, the underlying condition causing the ulcers should be identified and, if possible, treated. A prescription medication is available from pharmacists which both numbs the mouth and treats the ulcers. Before eating, the person should swish it around in the mouth and swallow it or spit it out. The ulcers themselves should be coated with a prescription medication containing codeine. If ulcers exist in the esophagus and stomach as well as in the mouth, it is necessary to swallow this medication. If the ulcers are caused by infection, the underlying infection should also be treated.

Enhancing Nutrition
If the patient is having a great deal of difficulty swallowing or digesting food, the physician will probably restrict some foods to prevent choking.* Some people may be limited to a liquid diet.

Caregivers need to be creative in working within the guidelines established by the physician. It is important to find food the person will like and can eat. Often foods from childhood, especially ethnic foods, are a favorite. Sometimes sweet foods, to which extra nutritional content can be added, are desired by the person. Some people, however, develop a complete aversion to sweet foods, in which case salty foods may be preferable. If the patient desires a particular food, whatever it may be, the caregiver should try to supply it and, if necessary, enhance it by adding powdered milk or a protein powder obtainable at a local health store, drugstore, or grocery store. Raw

---

* If there is an intestinal blockage, the caregiver needs to know if it is total or partial. A total blockage will prohibit any nutrition from being taken.

eggs should *not* be used in these preparations because of the danger of salmonella.

HELEN WRIGHT: The usual things wouldn't go down so well, so we would go back to childhood things, like macaroni and cheese. He found baby rice cereal very, very fine; that was something he could manage real well. But he would get tired of everything and it wouldn't taste right. He'd try. He knew that he needed vegetables; we knew he needed grain. He did his best. Near the end, he would try anything he could think of—anything that would come to his mind, I would try to make.

He couldn't take the Ensure.* That was frustrating to me, because everyone told me that would give him lots of nutrition. But he hated the taste. It was mainly that nothing tasted good. That was one of the most difficult things for me. I didn't want to push him; I didn't want to force him, but I was anxious. We would have sharp words occasionally because, you know, to stay alive you have to eat.

JOE STEAD: We tried everything to get her to eat but she wouldn't take anything. The last thing she ate was strawberry ice cream. She wanted strawberry ice cream, and I got it for her. She wanted her chocolate ice cream, and I got her that. I mushed it up a bit and put some milk powder in it. When the aide was here, she would make soup in the blender. I would try everything, anything I thought she would eat, anything. I saw her come to the table and take one mouthful.

Marijuana is a powerful and effective appetite stimulant because it reduces the nausea caused by some medications or the disease process. It is an illegal substance and therefore difficult to obtain, but authorities tend to look the other way if it is used for this purpose. For those who are concerned about the stigma of using an illegal drug, a physician can prescribe tetrahydrocannabinol (THC), which is the active ingredient in marijuana. A new FDA-approved pill, Marinol, contains THC and is helpful for nausea. The strength of pills is more difficult to tailor to the individual person's needs than is the inhaled marijuana, however.

There are several psychological approaches to enticing someone to eat. First, allow the person to have a choice in selecting the food. Second, stimulate the visual sense to encourage eating. For example, arrange the food attractively, on attractive dishes. The interestingly

* A brand of **nutritional supplement.**

shaped straws children use can make a liquid more interesting. Third, present the food in small amounts; large amounts are discouraging.

People who are taking mainly liquids can get extra nutrition by sucking on juice popsicles or juice made into ice chips. However, if the patient's mouth is ulcerated, juice may cause pain.

When swallowing becomes very difficult, liquids can be squirted into the mouth with a hypodermic syringe from which the needle has been removed. Squirt into the side of the mouth or cheek to prevent choking. A child's "sippy cup" with all but one of the holes covered by tape will allow the person to receive only a small amount of liquid and to hold the cup unaided. A straw cut in half can also be used for drinking.

Mouth Care
Good mouth care is essential in allowing the person to continue to take nourishment as long as possible. Helping the patient to brush the teeth and use mouthwash will help him or her feel fresh. When someone is no longer able to brush, the caregiver can clean the mouth and teeth with a Toothet, a small sponge on a stick. (A Toothet should *not* be used if the mouth is ulcerated. In that case, a swab dipped in cold water should be used with great care.) As death approaches and the person becomes dehydrated, keeping the mouth moist will be very important for comfort. (See the discussion of IV hydration in chapter 3.) The lips should be kept moist with lip balm.

The basics of nutrition for the dying are listed below.

Causes of poor nutrition:
lack of appetite, caused by the disease
poorly balanced diet
inadequate intake of calories
medication

Enhancing nutrition:
• Add powdered, nonfat dry milk or Carnation Instant Breakfast to soups, puddings, hot chocolate, milk shakes, casseroles, hot cereals, etc.
• Make homemade ice cream with cream and add nonfat dry milk or Carnation Instant Breakfast.

- Do not serve a hot liquid such as tea or soup before a meal because it fills the stomach and decreases the appetite.
- Substitute cream for milk whenever possible.
- Make juice ice chips and popsicles for sucking on.
- Provide nutritious snacks.
- Consult the hospital or hospice dietitian or write the American Cancer Society for specific recipes.

Causes of poor appetite:
inadequate exercise
loss of taste caused by chemotherapy, radiation treatments, or the disease process
change in sense of smell
fatigue
loss of sleep
medication

Stimulating the appetite:
- Encourage the person to do light exercise.
- Encourage the person to do range-of-motion exercises.
- Serve meals when the person is well rested and pain free.
- Serve 5–6 small meals a day.
- Give beer or wine before meals (with physician's permission).
- Serve favorite foods, often those of childhood.
- Keep portions small and arrange food appealingly.
- *Do not force the person to eat.*
- *Do not nag.*
- Season food with spices such as basil, tarragon, and lemon (but if there are mouth sores, avoid acids and spices).
- Use salt and sugar to season food, if the medical condition allows.
- Marinate meat in something sweet, such as wine or fruit juice.

Causes of nausea or vomiting:
the disease process
drug side effects
constipation
radiation treatments
chemotherapy

Dealing with nausea:
- After the person has vomited, offer water to rinse the mouth and clean the teeth to remove the taste.
- Remove the vomitus from the room quickly to eliminate smells.
- Keep the room well ventilated.
- Give small sips of herbal tea or black tea without milk.
- Serve small, frequent meals without liquids.
- Avoid overly sweet, greasy, or spicy foods.
- Provide dry foods such as crackers first thing in the morning.
- Use aromatic scents in conjunction with relaxation techniques when the patient senses a nausea attack coming on.
- If the nausea persists, consult a physician for medications that can alleviate it.
- Smoking marijuana has been shown to be extremely effective in relieving nausea; taking THC, the active ingredient in marijuana, is also effective.

Causes of painful or dry mouth:
medication, chemotherapy, or radiation treatments
dehydration
rapid breathing near death
decrease in fluid intake
malnutrition

Mouth care:
- Maintain oral hygiene; brush two times a day, three times if there is an infection.
- If the mouth is too painful to brush, clean with a cotton swab dipped in cool water.
- If the person is able to swish and spit out, use a solution of natural saline (2 tsp. salt in 1 qt. water) or baking soda (2 tsp. baking soda in 2 qts. water). Baking soda will make the mouth less hospitable to organisms.
- Toothets can be used to clean the teeth.
- Provide ice chips to suck, or fluids in small amounts (use straws to control flow of liquid so the person will not choke).
- Fruit juice popsicles can help, but some flavors may be painful for mouth sores.
- Provide soft, bland food, not spicy or hot, if ulcers are present.
- Tepid food is best; cool hot foods and warm cold foods.

- Do not use alcohol if mouth is inflamed. (Most commercial mouthwashes contain alcohol; check the label when buying one of these.)
- Remove dentures and soak them in mouthwash after meals and during the night.
- Encourage the wearing of dentures to retain jaw alignment, good appearance, and therefore self-esteem; when wearing dentures is painful, however, they should be removed.

Elimination

Either the disease process or the normal process of the body's shutting down which accompanies death eventually affects the body's abilities to eliminate waste products. Medications also affect the process of elimination. Dying people often become incontinent or constipated, or have diarrhea. Sometimes they experience several of these problems in sequence. For instance, diarrhea is often caused by constipation. These conditions must be evaluated by a physician or nurse *before* treatment is initiated.

Incontinence

Incontinence, losing control of bladder and/or bowels, can be deeply upsetting for the dying person. The loss of this control symbolizes loss of control over life. It is usually much more upsetting for the dying person than for the caregiver. Although cleaning up the "accidents" of the patient, especially if that person is a parent of the caregiver, can be the most forbidding aspect of caregiving for those who have never done it, it may quickly become routine for caregivers. It may, however, remain a problem for the dying person until the end.

> STAN CLARK: She was afraid she would lose bowel control in bed. Even up until five minutes before she died, she would repeatedly ask for the bedpan. We had to tell her it was O.K., but plainly it wasn't O.K. with her. It just wasn't. That was really hard for her.

Incontinence of bowel and bladder is a serious problem because of the effect on the skin. The skin of a dying, bedridden person is fragile because of inadequate nutrition and lack of exercise. Attempts should be made to keep urine and feces off the skin. The blue plastic pads used in hospitals to keep the bed dry should not be used next to the skin because they hold moisture close to the skin.

Pure cotton sheets should be next to the skin, with the blue plastic pad underneath. Although this makes it more difficult to change the bed, it will help prevent skin breakdown. For a terminally ill, incontinent woman, it is probably advisable to have an in-dwelling catheter inserted. Although a caregiver can be taught to perform intermittent catheterization, an in-dwelling catheter (which is a tube inserted through the urethra into the bladder and held in place by a small inflatable balloon) is less traumatic. A Foley catheter must be inserted and maintained by the home health or hospice nurse. Men can use a **condom** or **Texas catheter,** which can be fitted over the penis and is less intrusive than the in-dwelling catheter.

Constipation

Constipation can result from an inadequate diet, dehydration, the side effects of medication, immobility, or the body's shutting down in death. Constipation can be relieved by stool softeners, laxatives, enemas, or in extreme cases, disimpaction. The constipation can cause an oozing stool, which appears to be diarrhea. It is important to have this professionally evaluated so as not to mistreat.

To summarize, problems of elimination and ways in which the caregiver can deal with them are:

Causes of urinary incontinence:
disease pathology
dying process
urinary tract infection

Dealing with urinary incontinence:
- Have a commode next to the bed.
- Use a bedpan (or female or male **urinal**) for those who are bedridden.
- Limit fluids at night.
- Consider having a Foley catheter inserted. Do not tape the bag to the leg because this will irritate the skin.
- Check urine output. If a significant change occurs in output or color, call the hospice or home health nurse. (Shortly before death, urine output will become intermittent or cease altogether.)
- Make sure the urine in the bag does not back up into the catheter tube, for this would allow bacteria to enter the bladder and cause

an infection. To prevent backup, always keep the draining bag in a position lower than the person.

- When turning a patient, empty the drainage bag, then, *before turning,* place it on the side of the bed the person is being turned to.

Causes of diarrhea:
disease pathology
overuse of laxatives
side effects of medication
adverse drug reaction
constipation
infection

Dealing with diarrhea:
- Make sure person is not constipated: When was the most recent bowel movement? Was it normally formed? Is the abdomen distended?
- Give Kaopectate, Pepto Bismol, or Immodium A-D.
- When the person alternates between having diarrhea and having constipation, give Metamucil to bulk up the stool and encourage regular bowel movements.
- Increase fluids to prevent dehydration.
- Provide food low in fiber.
- Avoid spicy and fried foods.
- Avoid fat.
- Serve clear, warm—not hot—soups.
- Give crackers.
- Try the **"braty"** diet (bananas, rice, apple juice, dry toast, and yogurt).
- In extreme cases of diarrhea, **anal catheters** or **rectal tubes** can be used. Depending on the consistency of the feces and whether they are well contained, the bags can remain in place for 3–5 days.

Causes of constipation:
insufficient fiber
poorly balanced or inadequate diet
pain medication
inactivity

inadequate fluid intake
hypercalcemia or other metabolic causes

Dealing with constipation:
- Give stool softener. (As soon as a person begins taking a narcotic pain medication, a stool softener should be used.)
- Encourage exercise.
- Include fruit in the diet.
- Give a laxative if necessary.
- Insert a glycerin or laxative suppository.
- Administer an enema.
- In extreme cases, a nurse will have to disimpact the bowels. A caregiver can also be taught to do this.

If a patient complains of discomfort or has not had a bowel movement in three days (one week for someone who is close to death) or is oozing stool, call the nurse. (Even when a person is close to death and is not eating, the body continues to metabolize stored protein. This creates waste products, which must be eliminated.)

It is important to employ **universal precautions** when handling bodily fluids and waste. (See appendix E for further discussion.) It is possible to have HIV and not know it, thereby inadvertently putting the caregiver at risk.

Mobility and Falls

Although a few people in this book were able to walk and remained fully mobile until a few days before death, most suffered progressive impairment due to the disease process and general physical weakness. It is important to keep the dying person as mobile as possible, for mobility too implies adult status, and its loss is a blow to personal dignity and self-esteem. Dying children also prefer to be mobile. Two people in this book fought to regain their ability to walk despite their terminal diagnosis. Jim DeMott was successful, whereas Elizabeth Krolick was not.

The person's desire to walk should be encouraged, and assistance should be given as long as walking is possible. A cane or walker can be used to increase mobility. Problems arise when the person is no longer able to walk safely and begins to have falls. These can result from the advance of the disease or from the general weakness and confusion that can accompany the dying process.

HELEN WRIGHT: He continued to get up to go to the toilet. He didn't like to use the potty chair in the bedroom. So he would get up and I would say, "Now honey, I'll help you, I'll help you." I had helped him every time, every time, really—helped him to sit down, helped him to rise. But Wednesday night he got out of bed and got in there while I was asleep—I was dopey at this point with getting up so much at night— and he fell. He had a very hard fall, and I had such a hard time getting him up. He had another fall Thursday night, right in the middle of the night. He got up and didn't wait for me. I think he just didn't remember he was as weak as he was.

If the patient insists on walking despite the danger, the caregiver will have to consider tying him or her to the bed at night. This can be done with strips of gauze bandages, a folded sheet (see figure 4), or a **posey jacket**. Be careful not to apply these so tightly that they affect circulation. The problem of falls should not last long, for the weakness is progressive, and most people lose the ability to walk before death occurs.

To make a restraint system (see figure 4):

1. Fold a sheet into a long strip. Repeat with a second sheet.
2. Place one strip under the person's hips and the other on top of the waist.
3. Twist together or braid the loose ends of the strips on each side of the patient.
4. Tie the twisted sheets to the edge of the bed.
5. Tie securely, but allow for enough slack for the person to move.
6. Tie the hands down only if the person is trying to pull out lines or trying to hurt him- or herself.

The limbs should be kept mobile, regardless of whether the person can walk, to prevent the muscles from atrophying, which is an extremely painful condition. The hospice nurse or physical therapist can teach the caregiver to help the patient do range-of-motion exercises that are appropriate.

People in restraints should be checked every thirty minutes to an hour. Patients can make an effort to get free of the restraints and in so doing harm themselves. It is not safe to put someone in restraints and leave him unattended for the night.

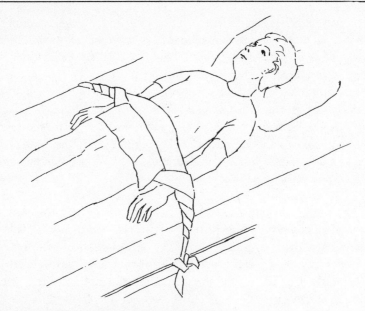

Figure 4. Restraint System, Using Gauze Strips

Transfers

Either because of the disease process or from the growing weakness that accompanies the dying process, most terminally ill people will eventually be unable to get in and out of bed or a chair by themselves. When this occurs, the caregiver or attendant will have to help. The caregiver *must* be trained to do this by a nurse or physical therapist. The training can be obtained in the hospital from the physical therapist or at home from the home health or hospice nurse. Pneumatic lifts, available from DME companies, permit one person safely to **transfer** even a larger person.

It is essential in all transfers that the caregiver take great care *not to strain her or his own back.* In addition, a transfer should not be attempted when the immobile person is extremely heavy; this can put the safety of both the dying person and caregiver in jeopardy. When the patient cannot bear weight, two people will be needed for the procedure. What follows is a list of the steps necessary to transfer from bed to chair. See figures 5 and 6 for an illustration of the technique.

1. If you are transferring the person to a wheelchair, *make sure the wheelchair wheels are locked.*

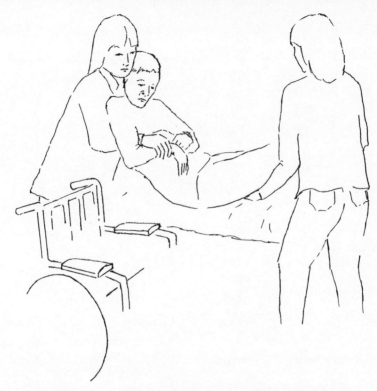

Figure 5. Beginning to Transfer Someone from Bed to Wheelchair

2. Evaluate the weight of the patient.
3. *Do not attempt a transfer* if there are doubts about the caregiver's ability to do it safely.
4. Lower the bed to the height of the chair to which the person is being transferred.
5. Stand at the head of the bed, behind the person.
6. Establish a good base of support, with the feet twelve to eighteen inches apart.
7. Stay close to the patient.
8. Slide your hands under the person's armpits from behind and reach forward to grasp his or her wrists.
9. Hold the patient close to your chest.
10. Have the helper slide his or her hands under the person's knees.
11. Using your leg and arm muscles rather than your back muscles, on the count of three, lift in unison.

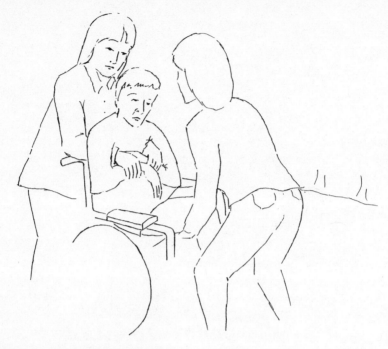

Figure 6. Completing the Transfer

12.   Step sideways and stand behind the chair.
13.   Gently lower the patient onto the chair.
14.   Arrange the person in a safe and comfortable position.

The same precautions must of course be taken when moving the patient from chair to bed.

Eye Care

In the advanced stages of some diseases, a person's ability to blink may be impaired. Sometimes the dying lose the ability to blink altogether. Artificial tears can help soothe the eyes. A warm washcloth placed over the eyes is also soothing; it should be wrung out first and changed frequently. To prevent damage if the blinking reflex is completely gone, eye patches can be placed over the eyes and removed when the patient needs to see.

Sleep

Dying people are often afraid to go to sleep—afraid they will never wake up. Some may actively resist sleep or take little catnaps throughout the day. Others sleep progressively more and more as death approaches and may eventually slip into a coma. Sleep cycle reversal, where the person sleeps during the day and is wakeful at night, can accompany many disease states. Lack of exercise makes restful sleep difficult. The dying person may be restless, agitated, and fearful.

Helping the person develop a regular pattern of sleep will maintain the sense of a functioning, stable household and serve to dispel the sense of crisis that can characterize the home at this time. A regular sleep pattern will reassure and calm the dying person as well as the caregiver. Sleep is more of a problem for the caregiver than for the patient, however. When sleep reversal makes it extremely difficult for the caregiver to sleep, daytime napping by the patient may be discouraged and often results in longer periods of sleep at night.

Routines help cue the body to prepare for sleep. A bedtime routine might include getting the bed straightened, turning the person, giving a back rub, medications, and a snack, playing relaxation tapes, and holding the person's hand until he or she is asleep. Warm milk, which acts as a sedative, can also help. If possible, the caregiver should try to sleep whenever the dying person sleeps, especially if the likelihood of being awakened during the night is high.

To avoid being wakened often to reassure the patient, place a large clock where the person can see it. Explain that the caregiver will return to check on the person at a certain time and ask not to be awakened until then, if possible. If the dying person is extremely fearful, he or she can sometimes be reassured by having the caregiver sleep in the same room, tying a string to the sleeping caregiver's hand, and giving the other end to the patient to hold.

When possible, dying people should be encouraged to exercise. Even sitting up in bed with the legs over the side helps. If possible, they should sit up in a chair several times a day. Isometric exercises, which involve contracting and then relaxing each muscle group in turn, can be done in bed.

In some cases medication can help people sleep. When cognitive impairment is involved, however, sleeping medication can sometimes have the opposite effect and cause agitation. As with pain medications, different combinations of medications and doses will have to be tried. Again, solving a sleeping problem with medication requires a good working relationship with the nurse and physician.

Here is a list of the causes and treatments of sleeplessness:

Causes of sleeplessness:
disease state
medications
lack of exercise
anxiety about death
depression
too many daytime naps

Treatment of sleeplessness:
• Encourage the person to do light exercises and isometrics.
• Have the patient sit in a chair.
• Have the person sit up in bed.
• Establish a bedtime routine.
• Provide only dim lighting at night.
• Maintain a quiet environment.
• Provide adequate ventilation.
• Serve a snack, but avoid fluids.
• Administer a gentle back rub.
• Decrease daytime naps.

Cognitive Impairment

Cognitive impairment refers to loss of the capacity to think clearly and includes loss of memory and the ability to recognize familiar people and places. Some people nearing death become cognitively impaired or agitated as a result of the disease process and the buildup of waste products in the body as it loses its ability to dispose of wastes. Cognitive impairment can also be a side effect of medication.

Progressive cognitive impairment can be a terrifying experience for the terminally ill, who frequently feel as if they are going crazy. Caregivers need to reassure the dying that this is part of the disease process. Although cognitively impaired people may inadvertently say some very funny things, it is imperative not to laugh, for this can distress them further, they don't understand the joke, and they can experience it as another frightening example of their insanity. Some laughter is inevitable; in such cases explaining to the person what exactly was funny can sometimes diminish the fear and anxiety created by the cognitive impairment.

Cognitive impairment can produce both auditory and visual hallucinations, in which the person perceives sights or sounds that are not actually present. Hallucinations can be extremely upsetting and frightening for the dying person and for the caregiver. For the well-being of both, it must be kept firmly in mind that hallucinations are produced by the disease process or as a side effect of the medications.

LAURA SWEET: A lot of weird things happened that I was really scared of. One night we were lying in bed and he said, "What is that noise?" I said, "I don't hear anything." He said, "Don't you hear anything? Be real quiet and we will hear these pages turning." I couldn't hear a thing. He said, "Yeah, someone is turning pages." So I said, "O.K., when you hear the noise squeeze my hand." He was squeezing my hand and I still couldn't hear anything. That was terrifying, really creepy. To appease myself and to make me get through the night I said, "Maybe it's just the morphine doing funny things to you." Maybe it was; that was scary.

Agitation

Agitation refers to fretful anxiety, fear, anger, and physical restlessness. The overall impression is of someone who is extremely upset and tense and uncomfortable. Agitation may have a physical cause, such as the inability to eliminate urine or feces. Possible physical causes should be investigated before agitation is treated with drugs. As one longtime hospice nurse said, "Always check the plumbing first," meaning "Make sure the person is able to eliminate." Inability to urinate or defecate can cause extreme discomfort. This symptom, as well as cognitive impairment, should be reported to the hospice nurse or physician and evaluated.

HELENA WOLF: The agitation was the impetus for putting him in the hospital. What I mean by agitation was his constant discomfort. Sometimes he talked appropriately, sometimes not, but he was constantly quite demanding. No matter how you moved him, it still hurt. You put the pillow here, you put the pillow there, it still hurt. Propping him up and supporting him and using heating pads—but he was still uncomfortable. The blanket was too tight, the blanket was too loose. It was clear that he never relaxed.

You had a sense of his being so wound up inside this body that basically worked not at all at that point that it became clear that this discomfort was so intense that you had to do something to help him. I think he could have stayed at home if we had catheterized him, which was basically all they did for him at the hospital. Clearly people could have done that; but no one suggested it, and I didn't know enough to ask.

It is difficult to achieve relief from agitation that does not have a physical cause. Tranquilizers, sleeping pills, pain medications, or alcohol (the person must be able to tolerate the burning sensation alcohol can produce in the mouth) can be used to produce a euphoric effect, but these substances can also cause depression. Some people argue that agitation results from the person's not having come to terms with death and that these substances will prevent the desired resolution by numbing the person psychologically. Conversely, some believe that people *not* receiving pain medications are denied the feeling of well-being that can accompany pain medications and that to deny those near death this sensation is cruel. To help resolve this conflict, consult with the nurse or physician about the causes and possible treatment of the agitation.

Administering Medication

Orally

As the body continues to shut down, the patient may refuse to take or be unable to swallow medication. If there is some degree of cognitive impairment and the caregiver has reason to believe that the person does not fully understand the implications of her or his actions, medication can be disguised in several ways. Some pills can be ground up and put in a strong-tasting liquid such as a dietary supplement. Check with the pharmacist to see if this is appropriate for a particular pill. Most medications come in alternative forms to facilitate administration. If the medication is given by syringe (without a needle) into the side of the mouth, the person cannot taste the medication as easily. One problem with administering medication in this way, however, is that it is difficult to determine how much of the dose has been received, especially if the person does not finish the liquid; but some medication is usually better than none at all.

A word of caution: The care of a dying person can be a frantic and intense experience. Be particularly careful not to leave medication open or easily accessible if young children are in the area.

By Injection

The idea of giving injections can cause considerable anxiety in people who have never done it before. In reality, though, it's a fairly simple process. However, the caregiver *must* be trained in the technique by a nurse. There are two kinds of injections which a caregiver may have to administer. The most common involves inserting a premeasured dose cartridge of medication into its hypodermic syringe. In the other, the caregiver must extract the dose by inserting the needle of the syringe into the rubber-topped medicine vial. Once the medication is in the syringe, these steps should be followed in giving the injection (also see figures 7, 8, and 9):

1. Pull back on the plunger to make sure it is full of medication.
2. Depress the plunger until all air is out of the cartridge. (Make certain a small quantity of liquid comes out the end of the needle.)
3. Choose a place for the shot: hip, thigh, or upper arm.
4. Feel for lumps, which indicate an injection was recently made in that spot; if lumps are present, choose another place.
5. Swab the site with alcohol.
6. For a subcutaneous injection, take a pinch of skin (see figure 7) and either poke or "wiggle" the needle. For an intramuscular injection in the arm (see figure 8), in the hip, or buttock (see figure 9), stretch the skin taut.
7. Push the needle all the way in.
8. Pull the plunger back slightly to check for blood. If blood enters the syringe, you have hit a vein and must try another spot.
9. Depress the plunger in a slow, steady movement taking no longer than three seconds.
10. Pull the needle out and press firmly on the site with a piece of cotton or tissue.
11. Dispose of the needle safely by dropping it in a needle disposal box provided by the DME company. If the medication was in a cartridge, remove the entire cartridge with the needle attached

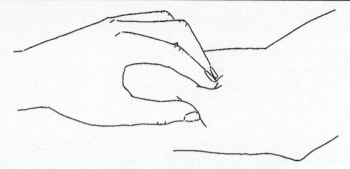

Figure 7. Preparing to Administer a Subcutaneous Injection

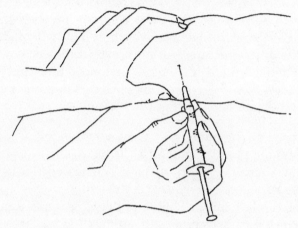

Figure 8. Administering an Intramuscular Injection in the Upper Arm

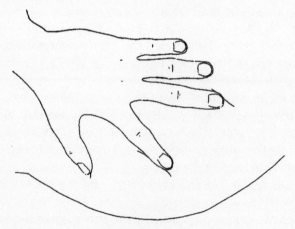

Figure 9. Preparing to Administer an Intramuscular Injection in the Hip or Buttock

and drop in the disposal box. If the medication was not in a prefilled cartridge, the entire syringe must be disposed of. *Do not recap the needle.* If a special disposal box is not available, drop the needle into a bottle of bleach with a screwable cap.
12. Anyone giving injections must take precautions. Always wear gloves when disposing of the needles.

Skin Patch
Morphine can be administered through a three-day **skin patch.** This form of morphine is called Fentanyl.

Sublingual
Pain medication in the form of a pill can be administered sublingually, which means under the tongue.

Intravenous Therapy
Intravenous therapy is generally available in the home. Many nurses and physicians prefer to deliver pain medication in this way when the patient requires larger doses and more continuous medication. The person should have a **venous access device**, which is an opening in a vein into which an **external catheter** or implanted **port** goes. The IV can then be inserted through this opening. This is better than a peripheral access (an access under the skin), in which the medication can infiltrate (gradually be released into) the surrounding tissue, a method that causes swelling and sometimes pain.

There are two main kinds of venous access devices: a **peripheral intravenous catheter (PIC line)**, which is an external catheter, and an implanted port. The external catheter can be directly connected to IV tubing. A port is like a rubber stopper inserted under the skin which gives access to a vein. Medication can be given by an injection into the port, and the person experiences no pain. An external catheter or a port must be inserted by a physician or surgeon, either in the hospital or on an out-patient basis. A PIC line allows medication to be inserted directly into the vein. It can be inserted in the home by a trained infusion therapist. A PIC line is best for an individual dying at home who does not yet have a venous access device, because it is easily inserted in the home setting.

With the access device, medication can be administered by a small pump. For pain medication, the pump allows continuous administration, and the patient is able to self-administer an extra dose, if necessary, for **breakthrough pain**. These pumps allow the alert person to exercise some control over this aspect of life and they can be used by the caregiver if the patient is not alert.

Some hospices refuse to deliver IV therapy in the home, in which case subcutaneous access is an acceptable alternative route.

Breathing Problems

Breathing problems can result from the disease and are an expected part of the dying process. Breathing may become irregular, or it may cease for periods and then start again. Caregivers should remain calm when it occurs. Breathing can also be very shallow.

Causes of breathing problems:
pathological process
nearness of death

Treatment of breathing problems:
• Increase the humidity in the room.
• Clean out mucus in the person's mouth and throat.
• Change the person's position and elevate the head 20°–30°.
• Administer or increase dose of oxygen.
• Keep the person's mouth and lips moist.

Oxygen

Oxygen is administered because of pathological damage to the lungs and is delivered through small tubes inserted into the nostrils. Oxygen is a colorless, odorless gas that is combustible. Do not smoke or have an open fire in a room where oxygen is in use. To ensure the dying person's comfort, pad the portion of the tube which goes over the ears, using gauze or cotton held in place by adhesive tape. Put Vaseline on the upper lip beneath the nostrils. To relieve the pressure from the nasal prongs, remove them occasionally. This can be done for 5–10 minutes without harm. Oxygen has a drying effect on mucous membranes, so make sure the oxygen unit has a humidifier.

Oxygen can also be used as a comfort measure to relieve anxiety about shortness of breath. There are certain criteria for ordering oxygen in hospice care. Making the patient more comfortable is an acceptable criterion whether or not the blood oxygen level is sufficient to require it.

Seizures

Seizures can occur when the dying person has a brain tumor, suffers from any one of a number of neurological diseases, or has a high fever. Caregivers need to ask the physician about the likelihood of a seizure so that they will be prepared if one occurs.

When a seizure occurs, *do not attempt to place anything between the patient's teeth.* This can injure the jaws or teeth. Turn the person's head to the side—the left side, if possible. Try to position the head lower than the feet (with a hospital bed, lower the head of the bed).

Causes of seizures:
brain tumor
neurological damage
fever
metabolic problems
decrease in oxygen

Treatment of seizures:
• Lay the person down to prevent falling.
• Turn the head to the side to keep airways open and facilitate vomiting, should it occur.
• If there are side rails on the bed, pad them to prevent injury.

Control of Pain

First, a dying person should not have to experience pain. Second, the medications given to relieve pain can be administered in such a way that the patient remains alert. This is the standard of care that caregivers must seek for the dying person. If it is not achieved, the caregiver should insist that the medical provider try to keep the patient pain free and mentally alert. With the expertise, technology, and medications available, home death should not be painful.

Even in the most painful kinds of cancers, such as bone cancer, the pain can be managed with the use of nonsteroidal anti-inflammatory drugs and antidepressants along with pain medication. Some physicians are not aware of advances in home-based therapy which ensure a pain-free death. To obtain this information for the physician, contact the cancer hotline (800-4-CANCER) for the name of the nearest oncologist and refer the physician to the oncologist for a consultation on pain medication. The caregiver can also contact the

Oncology Nurses Association, a nationwide organization with local branches, for information and referral.

Not all dying people are in pain. Fully one-third of the patients in this study required no pain medication, and two others required only episodic medication in the last days of life. When people do need pain medication, however, their need is intense. In urgency and seriousness, it surpasses any other problem caregivers will have to confront. *(Never use pain medication to control the dying person's behavior.)*

Many physicians and hospital nurses (though not hospital-based hospices, which provide excellent pain relief) continue to undermedicate for pain out of concern that the patient will become addicted. Dying people who are in pain do come to depend on the medication. However, if the dependency is for pain relief, it is not abuse. In fact, research shows that when people use narcotics for pain relief, they do not become addicted (Melzack 1990).

Part of the problem in undermedication for pain relief can be traced to the way the medication is administered. The standard method for administering pain medication is on a **pro re nata (PRN)**—as needed—basis. This means that the person must begin experiencing the pain *before* additional pain medication can be delivered. Because the pain associated with terminal illness can be so excruciatingly intense, controlling it may require giving a very large dose, and this can lead to mental clouding and other side effects, such as nausea.

An effective approach to pain tries to *prevent* it and helps the person lose the agonizing fear that it will return. Many people fear the return of pain more than they fear death. With this approach, morphine is given orally in a dose tailored to the person's needs every four hours, or more frequently if shorter intervals prove more effective for prevention. Because doses are frequent, they tend to be low, which reduces the chance of side effects. In one study, about 85 percent of cancer patients treated with this approach obtained satisfactory relief of their pain; the pain was either bearable or entirely gone (Melzack 1990).

There is no simple, straightforward assessment of pain. The intensity, quality, and frequency vary according to its location in the body and the sensitivity of the individual. A pain control strategy must be worked out for each individual. Unfortunately, this often must be accomplished by a process of trial and error. Certain drugs or combinations of drugs work for one person but not another. The same is true of dosage and frequency of dose. For some people, small, steady doses work better, and for others, large doses spaced further apart are effective.

As the person becomes sicker, the strategy for managing pain will have to be adjusted. The caregiver's observations will be invaluable here. Comatose people can experience pain and need medication. Signs that they are in pain include restlessness, picking at the skin, moaning, and groaning.

Assessment

The following assessment plan* can help the caregiver and dying person organize their observations to present to the physician or nurse, who can then develop a plan to treat the pain.

Pain Assessment Sheet
1. Location: Have the patient indicate where in the body the pain is located and whether it is deep or closer to the surface.
2. Intensity: The person should rate the pain on a scale of 0–5.
    0 = none
    1 = mild
    2 = discomforting
    3 = distressing
    4 = horrible
    5 = excruciating
3. Timing:
    Is the pain intermittent (that is, does it come and go)?
    Is it continuous?
    Does it have specific rhythms?
4. Quality: Describe the pain in the person's own words (for example, prick, ache, throb, pull, sharp).
5. How does the person express the pain? (Wincing, crying, moaning?)
6. What relieves the pain? Be as specific as possible.
7. What causes or increases it?
8. What effects does the pain have?
    Has accompanying symptoms (for example, nausea).

* Adapted from N. T. Meinhart and M. McCaffery, *Pain: A Nursing Approach to Assessment and Analysis* (New York: Appleton-Century-Crofts, 1983).

Interrupts sleep.
Suppresses appetite.
Decreases physical activity.
Affects relationships with others (for example, irritability).
Affects concentration.

Routes for Administering Pain Medication
Pain medication can be delivered by a number of routes:

oral
sublingual
rectal
intravenous
subcutaneous
intramuscular

The first choice for the administration of pain medication is the oral route, that is, pills or liquid taken by mouth. For the patient who has difficulty swallowing, however, there are effective alternatives.

Medication delivered sublingually is absorbed very quickly. For pain, a liquid medication with a high concentration of morphine can be placed under the tongue and can provide adequate pain relief.

Any drug—except time-release medication—which can be given orally can be administered rectally, in suppository form; the caregiver should first check with the physician or nurse that the medicine is not time released. A suppository can easily be made by crushing a pill, mixing it with margarine, shaping it, and freezing it. Storing the suppositories in the freezer makes insertion easier. A whole pill can also be inserted into the anus, but it is easier for the body to absorb the medication if it is in suppository form.

Intravenous medication can be delivered in several ways (see page 226, "Administering Medication") and is used when a patient cannot take the drug orally or needs it continuously. Morphine pumps are becoming increasingly easy to obtain, and they are extremely effective. The morphine is released directly into the body at a constant rate, and the person has the option of administering an extra dose when it is needed. The machine is programmed so that a fatal overdose is impossible. An infusion pump allowed Alice Clark to exercise a degree of control over this aspect of life.

STAN CLARK: She had this little machine to carry around that was filled with twenty-four hours of morphine. She was getting 30–34 milligrams of morphine an hour. We were always changing the rate. One of the things she could do was to give herself a bolus; this was totally under her control. It was a wonderful thing.

Pain medication that must be given continuously can also be delivered subcutaneously, that is, by an injection under the skin. This is also the best way of giving injections to someone who is emaciated. Subcutaneous injection is an efficient route when the veins have collapsed, making IV therapy extremely difficult or impossible.

An alternative route for injection is intramuscular, that is, into a muscle—usually of the upper arm, thigh, or buttock. Intramuscular injections are appropriate for medications that are given intermittently.

The use of pain medication creates side effects. As the health of the dying person becomes increasingly fragile, these cause more and more serious problems. One of the most difficult side effects to deal with is the tendency of narcotics to cause constipation and nausea.

Nonpharmaceutical Measures

Some kinds of pain can be relieved without medications; however, the pain of most forms of cancer usually requires drugs, often in heavy doses, especially toward the end of life. The nonpharmaceutical interventions described below can sometimes be effective throughout the stages of cancer pain and can also be used to relieve anxiety before a medication takes effect.

Relaxation techniques involving isometrics, massage, warm baths, visualization, and music may be useful in relieving pain. Relaxation, either active or passive, is especially effective in relieving muscular pain and painful breathing. When people are in pain, their first impulse is to tense the body to resist the pain. But tense muscles can make the pain worse, as many women who have experienced childbirth know (in fact, many of the relaxation techniques for pain relief are similar to those taught in childbirth classes). Thus relaxation techniques that reduce muscle tension can actually decrease the amount of pain experienced. Alice Clark used this training.

STAN CLARK: We had a procedure for calming down. It had to do with my talking her through deep and slow breathing and focusing on a calming activity to avoid panic attacks.

Isometric exercises produce muscular relaxation. Caregivers can assist patients by talking them through exercises. To do isometrics, the person first tenses the feet and holds for ten seconds, then releases. Next, the person tenses the calf muscles, then the thigh muscles, and so on, releasing each time after a count of ten. Gradually the muscle tensing moves up the body to the buttocks, stomach, hands, arms, shoulders, neck, and face. After the process is complete, the person determines if any part of the body remains tense and if so, concentrates on relaxing that part by imagining that he or she is "breathing" warm air into that area.

Giving someone a gentle massage is a good way both to relax the person and to keep the skin in shape. A gentle but firm massage on the back, face, arms, and legs can help in relaxation. Massages that exert pressure (such as the Swedish massage or Shiatsu) are probably not appropriate for the fragile body of a dying person. Alcohol-based lotions should be avoided because they dry the skin. Care should be taken in selecting a scent because many cancer and AIDS patients are very sensitive to smells.

Comfortably warm—not hot—baths can help people relax, and sometimes they relieve pain. This effect can be enhanced with a Jacuzzi set at low speed. Baths have certain drawbacks, however. The effort of getting into the tub may prove extremely exhausting for a fragile person and can sometimes be painful as well. Line the bathtub with towels in order to cushion the hard surface; alternatively, use a bath chair.

Transferring the dying person into the bath requires care. One or two people might have to stand in the tub to get the person safely in, and someone may have to sit down in the tub to hold the person up. In this case, the caregiver should simply sit down in the tub and hold the patient under the arms; the caregiver's knees provide additional support for the ill person. A piece of light clothing, such as an undershirt, may be worn by the patient if modesty is a consideration. The caregiver may want to wear a bathing suit.

Visualization refers to the process of systematically imagining scenes or incidents that help the individual symbolically to resolve problems. A famous example of visualization comes from cancer therapy, where the patient is encouraged to visualize his or her white blood cells attacking and destroying the cancer. Visualization can also work to relieve pain. The dying person remembers or imagines scenes that allow an escape from the painful present. Talking people through positive memories can help divert them from the pain and help them come to terms with their death.

Music can also be used as a means of helping to relieve pain. Because the sense of hearing often remains acute after all other senses have failed, music can be a powerful distraction and source of pleasure for the dying person.

The following are means of achieving relaxation without drugs. Caregivers and patients may find that one or a combination of them helps to relieve pain.

Isometrics
Massage
Warm baths
Visualization
Music

APPENDIX B

Additional Resources

General

To obtain information about local agencies or to lodge complaints concerning the conduct of an agency, write or call the department of public health, or the home care assembly or council, or the hospice association of the appropriate state.

For information and resources on managing pain in the home, contact the local branch of the Oncology Nurses Association, the local or state branch of the American Cancer Society, or call 800-4-CANCER for the name of the nearest oncologist. These resources can also be of assistance to professionals who might be unfamiliar with the particular needs of a specific patient. An oncologist is a specialist in the treatment of cancer. Unlike surgeons who also treat cancer, oncologists are experts in managing the symptoms and pain associated with terminal cancer. The oncologist can connect the caregiver and dying person with home-based support services in the area.

In many states the state department of health has information obtainable free of charge on choosing a home health care agency.

If professional help is not available or not satisfactory, caregivers may be able to receive training through the local Red Cross or the local community college, which may offer courses on home nursing.

Control of Pain

The American Pain Society is a pain control resource for professionals. It has chapters nationwide. Professionals can write or call their main office for a local contact.

American Pain Society
4700 W. Lake Avenue
Glenview, IL 60025
847-375-4715
(fax) 847-375-4777
http://www.ampainsoc.org

The Cancer Information Service will answer questions by telephone from patients, their families, the general public, and health care professionals. Printed materials are also available without charge.

Cancer Information Service
1-800-4-CANCER
http://www.nci.nih.gov/hpage/cis.htm

The National Cancer Institute houses and funds the Cancer Information Clearing House, which is an information service for organizations that use or develop cancer-related materials for the general public and for professionals. They provide information exchange either in the form of bibliographic services or in custom searches of data bases.

National Cancer Institute
Bethesda, MD 20205
301-496-7403

A useful handbook, published in 1987 for health care professionals providing care to the terminally ill is:

Domiciliary Terminal Care: A Handbook for Doctors and Nurses
by Dereck Doyle
Churchill Livingstone
New York

Another helpful handbook of this sort, published in 1989 is:

Palliative Care of the Terminally Ill
by J.F. Hanratty
Radcliffe Medical Press
Oxford

American Cancer Society
1599 Clifton Road, NE
Atlanta, GA 30329-4251
http://www.cancer.org

Living Wills

For information on the living will write to:

Society for the Right to Die
250 West 57th Street
New York, NY 10107

The Society for the Right to Die will send a living will form and a pamphlet describing the concept of the living will. It will still be necessary to check with an attorney or the local hospice to determine whether the living will is valid in the patient's state.

Another source for living wills is Concern for Dying. This is a non-profit educational group which provides living wills, durable powers of attorney, and information on euthanasia.

Concern for Dying
250 West 57th Street
New York, NY 10107
212-246-6962

The Living Will Center
http://www.rights.org/deathnet/LWC.html

Caregiving at Home

The American Association of Retired Persons offers a guide that may be of assistance: "A Path for Caregivers" (stock no. D1297). Send a written request including the stock number to:

AARP Fulfillment
1909 K Street, NW
Washington, DC 20049
http://www.aarp.org/caregive/home.htm
http://www.aarp.org/caregive/8-resour.htm

The California division of the American Cancer Society publishes a guide, "Caring for the Person with Cancer at Home," which is available from the local office of the society.

National Hospice Organization
1901 N. Moore Street, Suite 901
Arlington, VA 22209
703-243-5900
http://www.nho.org

Soros Foundation: http://www.soros.org/death.html

Last Acts
Robert Wood Johnson Foundation
P.O. Box 2316
Princeton, NJ 08543-2316
609-452-8701
(e-mail) mail@rwjf.org

For information about Yoga techniques of pain control, write to:

International Association of Yoga Therapists
4150 Tivoli
Los Angeles, CA 90066
213-306-8845

Another source for caregivers is *Thanatos: A Realistic Journal Concerning Dying, Death, and Bereavement.* For information write:

Thanatos
P.O. Box 6009
Tallahassee, FL 32314-9990

Nursing Homes

For information on nursing home care, the following sources can be of assistance:

The American Association of Retired Persons publishes a guide entitled, "Nursing Home Life: A Guide for Residents and Families" (stock no. D13063). For the address, see page 240, under "Caregiving at Home."

The Area Agencies on Aging were set up nationwide by the Older Americans Act. They serve as clearing houses for information on services to the elderly and sponsor research and demonstrations of innovative projects. To learn which agency is nearest, write to:

National Association of Area Agencies on Aging
600 Maryland Avenue, SE, Suite 208W
Washington, DC 20024

To obtain a copy of the free pamphlet, "Thinking about a Nursing Home: A Consumer's Guide to Long-Term Care," write, enclosing a self-addressed, stamped envelope to:

American Health Care Association
1201 L Street, NW
Washington, DC 20005
http://www.ahca.org

Suicide

For information on suicide write or call:

National Hemlock Society
P.O. Box 11830
Eugene, OR 97440
503-342-5748
http://www.hemlock.org/hemlock/general.html

Grief

For information on obtaining the services of a grief counselor write or call:

Association for Death Education and Counseling
National Office
638 Prospect Avenue
Hartford, CT 06105
203-232-4825

For information on services to help with grief write or call:

Grief Education Institute
2422 South Downing Street
Denver, CO 80210
303-777-9234

Family Services America
11700 West Lake Park Drive
Milwaukee, WI 53224
414-359-2111

The above organization publishes an annual directory of member agencies.

American Association of Marriage and Family Therapy
1717 K Street, NW, Suite 407
Washington, DC 20006
202-429-1825
http://www.aamft.org

The association offers a nationwide referral service of qualified therapists.

For information about *Bereavement: A Magazine of Hope and Healing,* write:

Bereavement Publishing
350 Gradle Drive
Carmel, IN 46032

To obtain a copy of the free brochure, "Grief Is Not a Sign of Weakness," write, enclosing a self-addressed, stamped envelope, to:

International Theos Foundation
322 Boulevard of the Allies, Suite 105
Pittsburgh, PA 15222
412-471-7779

For a copy of the booklet, "Holiday Help: Coping for the Bereaved," write, enclosing a check for $3.00, to:

Accord
1930 Bishop Lane, Suite 947
Louisville, KY 40218

Also see the journal *Thanatos*, address on page 241.

Gilda's Club
195 West Houston Street
New York, NY 10014
212-647-9700
(e-mail) mannheim@walrus.com

The Growth House
http://www.growthhouse.org

GriefNet
http://griefnet.org
(e-mail) griefnet@griefnet.org

Consumer health care information from the government:

http://www.healthfinder.gov

A large source of information:

http://www.npr.org/programs/death/resources3.html

Other web sites:

http://www.cancercareinc.org/patients/explorendoflife.htm
http://www.acponline.org/public/h-care/preface.htm

Pain Medications

The table below is not intended to be used as a guide for self-diagnosis. These medications are controlled substances and as such can only be given under the supervision of a physician.

Although the effective duration of the drug is listed, this should be seen as an average. People will differ in their response to pain medication according to the severity of their pain, its location, and their individual psychological make-up. Current thinking recommends that pain medication be given in smaller doses before the pain recurs. Establishing this preventive strategy tailored to the individual person's needs will require the expertise of a physician or nurse skilled in pain management (Melzack 1990). It is important to work with a health professional with expertise in pain management. Professionals without this expertise not uncommonly undermedicate for pain. Training in pain management is steadily becoming a standard part of physician training. Recently trained physicians should have this expertise. For intractable pain, consulting a pain management specialist is helpful.

Typically a dying person requiring analgesia will be started on a small to moderate dose, which will then be increased to maximize pain control with a minimum of side effects. The dosage range given below encompasses the typical starting and maintenance doses.

Table 2. Narcotic Analgesics for Severe Pain

Agent	Route	Normal Adult Dose	Peak Effect (hr.)	Duration (hr.)	Comments
Morphine (Roxanol, MS Contin)	IM	5–10 mg q 4 hr	0.5	6	Constipation, nausea, vomiting, and sedation are most common
	PO	10–30 mg q 4 hr	1.5–2	4–7	

Agent	Route	Normal Adult Dose	Peak Effect (hr.)	Duration (hr.)	Comments
	SR	30–120 mg q 12 hr	3–4	8–12	adverse effects. Do not crush SR tablets.
Codeine (various)	IM/SC/IV PO	30–180 mg q 4–6 hr	0.75–1.5 1.5–2	4–6 3–6	Sedation, stomach upset, constipation common. Tylenol w/codeine contains 325 mg Acetaminophen/ tablet. (Tylenol #3/#4 codeine content 30/60 mg per tablet.)
Oxycodone (Percocet, Percodan) Tylox	PO	10 mg q 3–4 hr	1	3–6	See morphine. Tylox contains 500 mg Acetaminophen/ capsule; Percocet contains 325 mg Acetaminophen/ tablet; Percodan contains 325 mg aspirin/tablet.
Levorphanol (Levo-Dromoran)	PO SC	2 mg q 2–4 hr	0.5–1	3–6	See morphine.
Hydromorphone (Dilaudid)	PO SC/IM	2–6 mg q 3–6 hr 1–2 mg q 4–6 hr	0.5–1 1–2	3–4 3–4	See morphine.
Oxymorphone (Numorphan)	IM/SC PR	1–1.5 q 3– 6 hr 5 mg q 4–6 hr	0.5–1 1.5–3	3–6 4–6	See morphine.

Agent	Route	Normal Adult Dose	Peak Effect (hr.)	Duration (hr.)	Comments
Meperidine (Demerol)	IM/SQ	50–150 mg q 3–4 hr	1–2	3–5	See morphine. Also causes CNS excitability.
Methadone (Dolophine)	PO IM/SC	2.5–10 mg q 3–4 hr	0.5–1.5	4–6	See morphine.
Fentanyl Transdermal (Duragesic)	Patch	25–100 mcg/ hr (change q 72 hr)	—	—	See morphine. Onset of analgesia takes 24 hrs. Effect persists 24–36 hrs upon removal of patch.
Propoxyphene (Darvon, Darvocet-N)	PO	32–65 mg q 4 hr (HCl salt) 100 mg q 4 hr (napsylate salt)	1.5–2	3–6	See morphine. Analgesic effect similar to tylenol w/codeine. Darvocet-N contains 650 mg Acetaminophen/ tablet.
Hydrocodone (Vicodin, Vicodin ES) Lortab	PO	5–10 mg q 4–6 hr	0.5–1	3–4	See morphine. Vicodin contains 500 mg Acetaminophen/ tablet; ES = 750 mg.

q=every; PO=oral; IM=intramuscular; IV=intravenous; SC=subcutaneous; PR=rectal; SR=sustained release (oral); CNS=central nervous system. Acetaminophen maximum dose per day should not exceed 4 gm.

Sources: U.S. Department of Health and Human Services, *Quick Reference Guide for Clinicians*, no. 9: *Management of Cancer Pain: Adults.* AHCPR Publication no. 94-0593, March 1994. *Caution:* Doses of aspirin and acetaminophen in combination with opioid/NSAID preparations must also be adjusted to the patient's body weight.

APPENDIX D

Sample Letters

Sample Letter to Physician

Dear Doctor,

As part of an ongoing effort to ensure high quality home care to cancer and hospice patients, we are currently investigating ways to support patients and their families and facilitate dignity and comfort in patients' final days.

Patients' families have sometimes experienced difficulties dealing with the necessary authorities after a patient's expected death in the home. As a result, these families have been subjected to needless additional distress at a time that is already very painful.

We have consulted local authorities' requirements for dealing with expected deaths in the home and believe that a letter from the attending physician, stating that death is imminent and that the patient and family have elected to allow the patient to die in the home, will prevent difficulties for the patient's family. This letter would be filed with the local authorities and should facilitate the necessary procedures at the time of death.

We therefore request such a letter from you and, for your convenience, have enclosed a letter indicating _____'s status and decision to die in the home. Please sign this letter and return it in the enclosed self-addressed, stamped envelope.

Sincerely,

Sample Physician's Letter

Date

Doctor's name
Address

TO WHOM IT MAY CONCERN:

(Patient's name) is presently under my care. (He/She) was diagnosed with (dx) in (month/year). (Patient's name)'s disease has progressed to a point at which no further treatment is warranted and (his/her) condition is terminal. In an effort to facilitate dignity and comfort in (his/her) final days, (patient and family or significant others) have elected (him/her) to die in the home. I am in support of (patient's name)'s decision and am willing to sign the death certificate in the event that this expected death does occur in the home setting.

Sincerely,

Caregiving and HIV

Introduction

Caring for someone dying of AIDS involves all of the strains we have so far discussed and some significant additional problems. Tragically, AIDS remains a highly stigmatized disease, which adds considerably to the suffering of both the person with AIDS (PWA) and the family and loved ones caring for the person. In this section we will address those issues and concerns in caregiving that are specifically related to AIDS. For a more detailed reference on AIDS caregiving, I suggest *The Guide to Living with HIV Infection,* by John G. Bartlett and Ann K. Finkbeiner, 4th ed. (Johns Hopkins University Press, 1998).

HIV infection and AIDS are frightening, because, until very recently in the United States and Europe, AIDS was almost invariably fatal. It remains so in the rest of the world. The high mortality rate combined with the fact that the first Americans to contract the disease were primarily members of stigmatized populations (homosexuals and IV drug users) have led some people to see the disease as punishment for moral transgressions. Diseases do not make moral judgments. Anyone can contract HIV. In countries where HIV is more prevalent than in the United States, it is transmitted heterosexually and women make up half of those infected. Everyone who contracts the disease deserves our concern and compassion.

Unfortunately, although we now know a lot about how AIDS is transmitted and its origin, people continue to be afraid of it and to isolate those who have the disease, including their family members. In part, this is a natural human reaction. People want to believe that this misfortune could not happen to them, so they say that the victim is somehow very different from themselves or that the victim did something to cause his or her own misfortune. This "blaming the victim" or depicting the victim as different from oneself is an all-too-human response to fear.

Although the caregiver may not approve of the way the PWA has lived life, it is important not to let those negative feelings affect the caregiving.

HIV infection/AIDS is now much more a chronic condition or disease and less a terminal diagnosis if it is identified early enough and appropriate therapy is begun. Combination antiretroviral therapy, especially with the addition of the protease inhibitor class of medications, has made a significant difference in forestalling an individual's development of AIDS and death. Death rates have decreased by over 40 percent nationwide since 1996, in large part because of these new therapies.

AIDS as defined by the Centers for Disease Control and Prevention certainly does not carry a prognosis of six months or less, unless the person has serious or numerous sequelae of the disease. It is not unusual for someone with AIDS to be labeled terminal and hospice-appropriate and then gradually (or in some cases suddenly) rally and live for a prolonged period because of taking antiretroviral medications for the first time. A terminal diagnosis should only be made after the person has been seen by an HIV specialist to ensure that all appropriate avenues of treatment have been taken. *Lazarus syndrome* refers to those persons who had AIDS and were given a limited prognosis, then got better, gained weight, and in some cases went back to work, mainly as a result of antiretroviral therapy.

Helping the Caregiver Cope

Social Stigma and Isolation

The caregiver of someone dying from AIDS must deal with strains and stresses not typically associated with caring for someone dying at home. Many PWA caregivers share the shame and guilt of their patient, and this makes it difficult for caregivers to know whom they can trust and talk to without being stigmatized. It is important, nonetheless, for caregivers to get support. The caregiver should be able to discuss openly issues in caring for the dying person—anger, fear, guilt, despair. The support person should have a history of being helpful and nonjudgmental and should be someone who will not disclose that the person cared for has AIDS.

In addition, there are now many support groups for PWAs and those who care for them. Often the PWA's physician or home care agency will know where such groups are located. A local HIV service agency will know how to get in touch with support groups. Support groups, which are strictly confidential, discuss ways the caregiver can cope. In support groups, people share their feelings as well as provide specific information about the disease and different therapies.

Social support is a key element in being able to care successfully for someone dying at home, but caregivers of PWAs often lack support because the stigma associated with the disease both frightens off potential supporters and makes the caregiver reluctant to seek support. These potentially negative feelings and conflicts will affect the caregiver's ability to provide care. Support groups can help caregivers get in touch with their own anxieties and conflicts about AIDS as well as help them understand what a potential supporter might be feeling. The caregiver can assist the supporter by addressing the supporter's fears. For example, if the caregiver could say to the dying person's friend, "I know this might be upsetting, and you are afraid you might get AIDS, but you won't if you're careful, and I could really use your help." Even so, some people will be unable to help. This doesn't necessarily mean the person does not care about the dying person or the caregiver. (See chapter 4 for a more detailed discussion of social support.)

If caregiving begins to affect the caregiver's job, possibly requiring a cutback at work, it may help to say that the spouse/child/friend/partner is "very sick and needs me." If there are any doubts about how the employer will react or if they will keep the knowledge in confidence, it may not be appropriate to disclose that the person has AIDS. Whom to tell and how much to tell will be an ongoing concern in AIDS caregiving as the caregiver balances a need for support against the prejudices and responses of others toward AIDS.

Fear of Transmission

Despite popular hysteria, HIV is not easy to get. Caregivers need to educate themselves about the disease and how it is transmitted. By instituting proper infection-control procedures, the risk of contracting the disease in caregiving can be eliminated.

Despite the relatively simple steps to prevent infection, people remain frightened of contracting the disease. Talking with professionals involved in the PWA's care (e.g., the physician, nurse, home care personnel) can help alleviate these fears through information and further education. It is helpful to establish a relationship with a health care professional who can provide information about specific concerns in HIV transmission.

Neurological Changes as a Result of HIV Infection

One of the most challenging aspects of caring for someone with AIDS is coping with the neurological changes that the disease may cause. Over one-third of people with AIDS suffer cognitive impairment. Memory loss and a decreased ability to concentrate are among the first signs of HIV infection in the central nervous system. The impact on the nervous system ranges from very mild to severe, depending on the specific course of each PWA's disease. A caregiver must be prepared to deal with the mental changes in the PWA. A high dose of AZT has been shown to help this condition in some circumstances so the caregiver should discuss its possible benefit with the physician.

Cognitive problems are among the most difficult to cope with because they seem to change the patient into a different person. Erratic behavior (sometimes violent) and personality changes can leave the caregiver feeling that he doesn't know whom he is caring for. It is important to remember that behavioral changes are just as difficult for the patient and very frightening, because the PWA can think that he or she is going mad. Continue to remind the person that the changes are the result of the disease, not madness.

Cognitive changes can create specific caregiving problems, especially if the PWA begins to forget or refuses to take medication. Appointments, meals, and bills are also forgotten, as well as safety measures such as turning off the stove. If forgetfulness progresses, the caregiver needs to pay attention to the PWA's safety. The person may not be able to be left alone, and the environment should be kept clear of potential hazards, such as an open stairwell.

It can be extremely frustrating to deal with cognitive and behavioral changes. Sometimes it seems as if the PWA is deliberately acting strangely or creating a disruption in order to make things difficult for the caregiver. Remembering that these actions are caused by the disease can reduce a caregiver's anger and frustration. Seeking reassurance and information from professional caregivers is an important resource for dealing with these changes.

Impact on Children

Some caregivers will also have to care for the PWA's children. Children are exposed to and pick up the many popular fears and misconceptions about AIDS. They may have a very skewed understanding of the disease and a negative image of people who have it. In addition, they may worry that the caregiver will contract the disease and that they will lose the caregiver, too; they may also fear for their own lives. The caregiver, with the help of a health care professional, can teach the children about safely interacting with the PWA, thus reducing their fears about transmission. Children will need help in sorting out their feelings and fears, as well as advice on dealing with their friends, most of whom will also share their fears and misconceptions. In some cities, support groups for families of PWAs are available to help children cope with having a family member stricken with AIDS.

Uncertainty

The uncertainty about the disease process, length of caregiving (see chapter 5), and changes that the PWA will undergo is common to all diseases, especially those perceived to be terminal. Although it is important to realize that the course of HIV infection is different in every person, there are some relatively common criteria that assist the caregiver in anticipating needs and concerns of the PWA. Learning about HIV infection and establishing relationships with other AIDS caregivers and with the doctors and nurses involved in the PWA's care can help alleviate this uncertainty.

Infection Control Precautions for the Home Setting

The risk of HIV transmission from sharing a household with a PWA is negligible, and those documented cases where infection *did* occur were via the blood-to-blood route, e.g., two teenage boys sharing the same razor. The three routes of transmission are:

1. *Sexual Contact* (with the exchange of body fluid, e.g., semen, vaginal secretion)
2. *Blood to Blood* (includes heroin users sharing the same needles, and hemophiliacs and others infected with HIV via blood transfusion)
3. *Pregnancy/Birth* (one in three or four babies born to an HIV infected mother will eventually be HIV+ themselves. Note: new research

has established that if the mother takes AZT during her pregnancy, it dramatically reduces the risk of transmission to the fetus)

HIV is contained in some body fluids in greater concentration, e.g., blood, semen, breast milk, than in others, e.g., tears and saliva. To pass HIV infection to another person, HIV must travel from one person's body into another person's bloodstream in a high enough concentration to infect them. Among the factors known to affect transmission are the presence of open genital lesions during intercourse and the concentration of HIV in body fluid transmitted from the HIV infected person to the noninfected person. Studies of health care workers sustaining needle pokes and injuries from needles used with HIV infected persons show that only one in approximately two hundred and fifty of the health care workers will go on to test HIV+ from that one exposure.

HIV is not transmitted by shaking hands, sharing a bathroom or eating utensils, living in the same household, hugging someone, or kissing them on their cheek.

There is no risk associated with simply living in the same household or working in the same office as someone who has HIV. To date there have only been two recorded cases of home caregivers contracting the disease, and they took absolutely no precautions against infection. A few simple, commonsense precautions will ensure that the caregiver and other household members do not contract the virus.

(The following list is adapted from *The Guide to Living with HIV Infection*, chap. 2, "Preventing Transmission of HIV . . .").

Handwashing. This is the most important way to prevent the spread of any infection, not just HIV. Wash hands under hot water with soap or germicide for at least ten seconds. Rinse thoroughly and then dry the hands.

Gloves. Wear gloves if your hands have any cuts or torn cuticles. Wear gloves to handle blood, feces or urine, or to clean open sores. Wear gloves to clean surfaces or clothes soiled by blood, feces, or urine. Most health care professionals use latex gloves for this purpose. After using, wash the gloves and dispose of them in a container, like a trash can, that is lined with a plastic bag.

Disinfectants. Disinfectants like common household bleach should be used to clean surfaces contaminated by fluids containing the virus. A solution of one part bleach and nine parts water (1:10) is sufficient to kill the virus. This solution should be left on surfaces for ten minutes, then wiped off. Gloves should be used when cleaning with disinfectants to protect the skin. The bleach solution should be properly stored and labeled to prevent accidentally confusing it with water.

Dishwashing. The PWA can use the same dishes as other household members. The dishes should be washed in the dishwasher or with hot soapy water.

Laundry. Laundry should be washed with detergent in hot water. One-third cup of bleach added to the wash will ensure that it is disinfected, but this can damage some fabric. Fabric soaked with blood or bodily fluids should be presoaked and washed separately. Dry cleaning disinfects any fabric.

Cuts and other injuries. If the caregiver or PWA has an open cut or bleeding sore, the blood should be wiped clear and the area dabbed with alcohol (70 percent isopropyl).

Blood spills. If blood, including menstrual blood, is spilled on a surface, it should be wiped clean with disposable cleaning rags by someone wearing disposable gloves. The area should be cleaned with a disinfectant in either a 1:10 or a 1:100 dilution. Mops or other cleaning utensils used in cleaning the spill can be cleaned with soap and water.

Disposal of waste. Liquid waste that may have HIV in it can be poured down the toilet or sink. The sewer system has the means to treat contaminated waste.

Soiled materials such as bandages, sanitary napkins, disposable gloves, or cleaning cloths should be thrown away in a trash container lined with a plastic bag.

Sharp instruments such as needles, syringes, or used razor blades should be disposed of in a metal container such as an old coffee can. Some health departments recommend adding bleach to the can.

Home Health Care Needs of Adults with HIV

Many of the home care needs of the PWA are the same as those of any person with a terminal illness. Perhaps the most significant problems associated with HIV are weakness, lethargy, shortness of breath, and general fatigue. This set of problems both exacerbates and is caused by poor nutritional status. Malnutrition is a disease process that occurs along with AIDS and is curable and often preventable. A PWA can sometimes be so tired that he or she cannot eat, which in turn increases the fatigue.

Fatigue may be combined with cognitive problems, which make it more difficult to perform simple daily activities such as food preparation, cleaning, laundry, shopping, bathing, taking medication, or climbing stairs. As the PWA becomes sicker, it may also be difficult to walk, dress, use the toilet, or eat unassisted.

There are specific interventions to help the PWA conserve strength.

Attention to nutrition. Because the PWA may not have the energy to eat properly, assistance is needed in the provision and preparation of food. It may also be necessary to remind the PWA to eat once the food is prepared. (See Appendix A for more detailed discussion of nutrition.)

Conserving strength. Lethargy and fatigue are part of the disease and even good nutrition will not completely solve these symptoms. It is thus important to conserve the PWA's energy and strength. Activity should be balanced with rest. When needed, the caregiver or other helper should assist with household chores and basic self-care. A wheelchair should be used whenever the PWA may have to stand or walk for a sustained period, such as a doctor's visit or church service. If possible, the PWA should sleep on the first floor to avoid climbing stairs. As the PWA becomes weaker, a beside commode can be used.

Supervision of the cognitively impaired. As noted earlier, it may be necessary to remind the PWA to take medications and remember appointments. Further, the caregiver should attend to safety issues in the home. If cognitive problems and the resulting behavior become severe, the caregiver can consult *The 36-Hour Day,* by Nancy L. Mace and Peter V. Rabins, 3rd ed. (Johns Hopkins University Press, 1999). This book helps a caregiver cope with the challenge of caring for someone with dementia, providing a wealth of suggestions for caring for the cognitively impaired.

It is important to remember that the PWA is not acting willfully; instead, the disease is causing the disruptive behavior.

Pain

Common types of pain in HIV infected individuals include headache, chest pain, and pain caused by peripheral neuropathy. Headache is related to the virus itself or an associated condition such as meningitis or an adverse reaction to a medication. Most chest pain is related to an opportunistic infection, especially *Pneumocystis carinii* pneumonia (PCP) or candidal esophagitis. Peripheral neuropathy is perhaps the most common cause of chronic pain in those with advanced HIV infection. It is related primarily to the virus itself and usually affects the lower extremities, especially the feet. It has a negative effect on quality of life, making walking difficult and reducing energy. Traditional pain medications and modalities often do not assist this neuropathic or "nerve" pain, and other options are utilized, such as antidepressants (for example, Elovil) or antiseizure medications (like Neurontin). In addition, these patients invariably require an opioid, like morphine or Duragesic, because of the severity and chronicity of their pain. Prolonged walking or standing and tight-fitting socks or shoes are to be avoided, and using a wheelchair may be necessary when outside the home. Other sources of pain in persons with AIDS include herpetic pain from the ulcers caused by the herpes simplex or herpes zoster viruses and abdominal pain related to infection or medication.

Rights of HIV Infected Patients

Unfortunately, because of the stigma associated with HIV, some health care professionals will try to avoid treating people with HIV or will treat them in a substandard and inappropriate fashion. It is important to be aware of what the patient's rights are and to insist on those rights. According to the 1990 Americans With Disabilities Act it is illegal to refuse treatment to a patient simply because the patient has AIDS.

The following discussion of the patient's rights in hospitals is adapted from *The Guide to Living with HIV Infection*. (See chapter 2 of this book for a detailed discussion of dealing with hospital bureaucracy and acting as a patient advocate.)

1. Any patient has a right to be treated with respect. This includes getting answers to questions about medical condition and care. If hospital personnel are not doing this, the PWA or his representative should complain to the hospital administration.
2. Any patient has a right to expect that medical records and facts about their condition be kept private and confidential. This is an especially sensitive issue for people with AIDS. The diagnosis of

AIDS and related conditions must be entered into the patient's medical record. These records are available to all who need to see them, such as the physicians and nurses involved in the patient's care. The information is also sent to the Centers for Disease Control, and some states require that all cases be reported to the state department of health. Hospitals should restrict access to the records to only those who need to see them. It is not appropriate to post on the door or above the patient's bed that the person has AIDS.

3. A person has the right to participate in decision making concerning medical treatment. Medical conditions should be explained as clearly as possible. The PWA should be told what the procedures or treatment involve and what the possible risks or benefits are.

4. Patients have a right to be interviewed and examined in a private setting. They can ask anyone not involved in their care to leave. They also have the right to restrict visitors to their room. This can be accomplished by telling the physician or nurse responsible for their care.

5. Mentally competent patients can reject any form of treatment offered. Heroic life-sustaining measures at the end of life are the most frequent types of treatment that people reject. It is important to consider whether or not the patient wants to be put on life-support systems or to have heroic measures used to prolong life before these measures are needed. Advance directives or a living will can tell the physician in charge as well as the patient's family members about the patient's wishes in regard to specific forms of treatment. The laws concerning a living will vary from state to state. Many hospitals have information on living wills. (See appendix B for additional sources of information.)

6. The patient has a right to refuse to participate in any research program, and this should not affect access to treatment or the quality of treatment received.

7. Patients can communicate with whomever they wish. This includes physicians, lawyers, and members of AIDS advocacy groups.

8. A person may leave the hospital against the advice of the physician. To do so, the patient or the patient's legal representative must sign a form called a "Discharge Against Medical Advice." This action may sever the physician-patient relationship. In some states patients with certain contagious diseases, which are possibly infectious to others, may be restrained from leaving the hospital. This is not likely to be an issue for people who are dying.

9. People may not be transferred from one facility to another without a full explanation of the need for the transfer and any alternatives to the transfer. The receiving institution must also agree to accept the transfer.
10. When a patient is discharged from the hospital, the patient has a right to information about continuing health care requirements, which include medications, follow-up visits, nutrition, and limitations on activity.
11. A person has a right to ask about any financial charges by the hospital, the clinic, and the physician and to ask for various options for payment.

End-of-Life Decisions

Chapter 7 contains a detailed discussion of end-of-life issues, but there are some issues that mainly concern PWAs that will be discussed here.

Some families of PWAs involved in same-sex relationships will not have come to terms with the PWA's lifestyle and may not accept the PWA's partner or friends. Families may refuse to include the partner in decisions regarding the PWA's medical care or end-of-life plans. To help prevent emotionally draining and potentially traumatic conflicts, it is important that the PWA specify in advance who is to make decisions for the PWA in the event that the person can no longer do so, and what kind of end-of-life arrangements the PWA desires.

This can be done by drawing up a **durable power of attorney for medical care** and a **durable power of attorney for financial matters.** The patient specifies which powers to include in the durable power of attorney. The person who holds the power of attorney for financial matters cannot make medical decisions, although the patient can specify that the same person hold both powers of attorney.

The durable power of attorney for medical care takes effect when two physicians, one the patient's physician-of-record, decide that the patient is no longer capable of understanding or communicating decisions about his own health. The person who holds the durable power of attorney then assumes the powers identified in the document and must honor the patient's wishes specified in the document. Typically, this gives the person with the durable power of attorney the authority to refuse life-prolonging treatment for the patient. It may also include the power to make decisions about burial if the PWA dies.

The durable power of attorney must be signed by the person giving the power of attorney, the person to whom the power of attorney is given, and two witnesses who are not interested parties. Some states require that the document be notarized. Lawyers and hospital legal offices can provide models for such documents.

A copy should be kept by the person assigning the power of attorney and by that person's lawyer or some other responsible party. It remains in effect as long as the person is incompetent.

The durable financial power of attorney takes the same form as the medical power of attorney. It can assign the power to make decisions in the areas of business or banking, which includes signing checks. The power can be broad or very narrow.

This power of attorney also takes effect only when two physicians declare the person assigning the power of attorney incompetent, which means that the PWA is incapable of understanding and communicating financial decisions. As with the durable medical power of attorney, it remains in effect as long as the person is incompetent.

Funerals can be an especially difficult and sensitive issue for PWAs, their families, and loved ones. Caregivers should make serious efforts to accept or come to terms with their loved one's lifestyle. If the family and the partner of the dying person cannot come to terms, perhaps two funerals are needed. If possible the dying person should state their wishes for two funerals.

(This appendix was written with the assistance of Gerald Burns, RN.)

APPENDIX F

Michigan Dignified Death Act

Public Act 594 of 1996
Adds Part 56a and amends sections 16221 & 16226

333.5651 *Short title of part.*

Sec. 5651. This part shall be known and may be cited as the "Michigan dignified death act".

History: Add. 1996, Act 594, Eff. Mar. 31, 1997.

333.5652 *Legislative findings.*

Sec. 5652. (1) The legislature finds all of the following:

(a) That patients face a unique set of circumstances and decisions once they have been diagnosed as having a terminal illness.

(b) That published studies indicate that terminally ill patients fear that in end-of-life situations they could receive unwanted aggressive medical treatment.

(c) That terminally ill patients are often unaware of their legal rights, particularly with regard to controlling end-of-life decisions.

(d) That the free flow of information among health care providers, patients, and patients' families can give patients and their families a sense of control over their lives, ease the stress involved in coping with a terminal illness, and provide needed guidance to all involved in determining the appropriate variety and degree of medical intervention to be used.

(2) In affirmation of the tradition in this state recognizing the integrity of patients and their desire for a humane and dignified death, the Michigan legislature enacts the "Michigan dignified death act". In doing so, the legislature recognizes that a well-considered body of common law exists detailing the relationship between health care providers and their patients. This act is not intended

to abrogate any part of that law. This act is intended to increase terminally ill patients' awareness of their right to make decisions to receive, continue, discontinue, or refuse medical treatment. It is hoped that by doing so, the legislature will encourage better communication between terminally ill patients and health care providers to ensure that a terminally ill patient's final days are meaningful and dignified.

History: Add. 1996, Act 594, Eff. Mar. 31, 1997.

333.5653 Definitions.

Sec. 5653. (1) As used in this part:

(a) "Health facility" means a health facility or agency licensed under article 17.

(b) "Medical treatment" means a treatment including, but not limited to, palliative care treatment, or a procedure, medication, surgery, diagnostic test, or hospice plan of care that may be ordered, provided, or withheld or withdrawn by a health professional or a health facility under generally accepted standards of medical practice and that is not prohibited by law. As used in this part, "hospice" means hospice as defined in section 20106 of the public health code, Act No. 368 of the Public Acts of 1978, being section 333.20106 of the Michigan Compiled Laws.

(c) "Patient" means an individual who is under the care of a physician.

(d) "Patient advocate" means that term as defined in section 496 of the revised probate code, Act No. 642 of the Public Acts of 1978, being section 700.496 of the Michigan Compiled Laws.

(e) "Patient Surrogate" means the parent or legal guardian of a patient who is a minor or a member of the immediate family, the next of kin, or the legal guardian of a patient who has a condition other than minority that prevents the patient from giving consent to medical treatment.

(f) "Physician" means that term as defined in section 17001 or 17501.

(g) "Terminal illness" means a disease or condition due to which, in the opinion of a physician, a patient's death is anticipated within 6 months after the date of the physician's opinion.

(2) Article 1 contains general definitions and principles of consultation applicable to all articles in this code.

History: Add. 1996, Act 594, Eff. Mar. 31, 1997.

333.5654 Recommended medical treatment for terminal illness; duty of physician to inform orally; requirements.

Sec. 5654. (1) A physician who is recommending medical treatment for terminal illness to a patient who has been diagnosed as having a terminal illness shall do all of the following:

(a) Orally inform the patient, the patient's patient surrogate, or, if the patient has designated a patient advocate and is unable to participate in medical treatment decisions, the patient advocate acting on behalf of the patient in accordance with section 496 of Act No. 642 of the Public Acts of 1978 about the recommended medical treatment for the terminal illness and about alternatives to the recommended medical treatment for the terminal illness.

(b) Orally inform the patient, patient surrogate, or patient advocate about the advantages, disadvantages, and risks of the recommended medical treatment and of each alternative medical treatment described in subdivision (a) and about the procedures involved in the recommended and each alternative medical treatment.

(2) A physician's duty to inform a patient, patient surrogate, or patient advocate under subsection (1) does not require the disclosure of information beyond that required by the applicable standard of practice.

(3) Subsection (1) does not limit or modify the information required to be disclosed under sections 5133(2) and 17013(1).

History: Add. 1996, Act 594, Eff. Mar. 31, 1997.

333.5655 Recommended medical treatment for terminal illness; duty of physician to inform orally and in writing; requirements.

Sec. 5655. In addition to the requirements of section 5654, beginning 120 days after the effective date of the amendatory act that added this part, a physician who is recommending medical treatment for terminal illness to a patient who has been diagnosed as having a terminal illness shall, both orally and in writing, inform the patient, the patient's patient surrogate, or, if the patient has designated a patient advocate and is unable to participate in medical treatment decisions, the patient advocate, of all of the following:

(a) If the patient has not designated a patient advocate, that the patient has the option of designating a patient advocate to make medical treatment decisions for the patient in the event the patient is not able to participate in his or her medical treatment decisions because of his or her medical condition.

(b) That the patient, or the patient's patient surrogate or patient advocate, acting on behalf of the patient, has the right to make an informed decision regarding receiving, continuing, discontinuing, and refusing medical treatment for the patient's terminal illness.

(c) That the patient, or the patient's patient surrogate or patient advocate, acting on behalf of the patient, may choose palliative care treatment including, but not limited to, hospice care and pain management.

History: Add. 1996, Act 594, Eff. Mar. 31, 1997.

333.5656 Standardized written summary; development; publication; contents; availability to physicians.

Sec. 5656. (1) Within 60 days after the effective date of the amendatory act that added this part, the department of community health shall develop and publish a standardized, written summary that contains all of the information required under section 5655.

(2) The department shall develop the standardized, written summary in consultation with appropriate professional and other organizations. The department shall draft the summary in nontechnical terms that a patient, patient surrogate, or patient advocate can easily understand.

(3) The department shall make the standardized, written summary described in subsection (1) available to physicians through the Michigan board of medicine and the Michigan board of osteopathic medicine and surgery created in article 15. The Michigan board of medicine and the Michigan board of osteopathic medicine and surgery shall notify in writing each physician subject to this part of the requirements of this part and the availability of the standardized, written summary within 10 days after the summary is published.

History: Add. 1996, Act 594, Eff. Mar. 31, 1997.

333.5657 Availability of form to patient, patient surrogate, or patient advocate; compliance with § 333.5655; placement of signed form in patient's medical record; signed form as bar to civil or administrative action.

Sec. 5657. (1) If a physician gives a copy of the standardized, written summary made available under section 5656 to a terminally ill patient, to the patient's patient surrogate, or to the patient's patient advocate, the physician is in full compliance with the requirements of section 5655.

(2) A physician may make available to a terminally ill patient, to the patient's patient surrogate, or to the patient's patient advocate a form indicating that the patient, patient surrogate, or patient advocate has been given a copy of the standardized, written summary described in section 5656 and received the oral information required under section 5654. If a physician makes such a form available to a terminally ill patient, to the patient's patient surrogate, or to the patient's patient advocate, the physician shall request that the patient, patient's patient surrogate, or patient advocate sign the form and shall place a copy of the signed form in the patient's medical record.

(3) A patient, a patient's patient surrogate, or a patient advocate who signs a form under subsection (2) is barred from subsequently bringing a civil, or administrative action against the physician for providing the information orally and in writing under section 5655 based on failure to obtain informed consent.

History: Add. 1996, Act 594, Eff. Mar. 31, 1997.

333.5658 Prescription of controlled substance; immunity from administrative and civil liability.

Sec. 5658. A physician who, as part of a medical treatment plan for a terminally ill patient, prescribes for the terminally ill patient a controlled substance that is included in schedules 2 to 5 under part 72 and that is a narcotic drug is immune from administrative and civil liability based on prescribing the controlled substance if the prescription is given in good faith and with the intention to treat a patient with a terminal illness or alleviate the patient's pain, or both, and all of the following are met:

(a) The prescription is for a legitimate legal and professionally recognized therapeutic purpose.

(b) Prescribing the controlled substance is within the scope of practice of the physician.

(c) The physician holds a valid license under article 7 to prescribe controlled substances.

History: Add. 1996, Act 594, Eff. Mar. 31, 1997.

333.5659 Life insurer, health insurer, or health care payment or benefits plan; prohibited acts.

Sec. 5659. A life insurer, a health insurer, or a health care payment or benefits plan shall not do 1 or more of the following because a terminally ill patient, the patient's patient surrogate, or the patient's patient advocate has made a decision to refuse or discontinue a medical treatment as a result of information received as required under this part:

(a) Refuse to provide or continue coverage or benefits to the terminally ill patient within the scope and level of coverage or benefits of an existing policy, certificate, or contract.

(b) Limit the amount of coverage or benefits available to a terminally ill patient within the scope and level of coverage or benefits of an existing policy, certificate, or contract.

(c) Charge the terminally ill patient a different rate for coverage or benefits under an existing policy, certificate, or contract.

(d) Consider the terms of an existing policy, certificate, or contract to have been breached or modified.

(e) Invoke a suicide or intentional death exemption or exclusion in a policy, certificate, or contract covering the terminally ill patient.

History: Add. 1996, Act 594, Eff. Mar. 31, 1997.

333.5660 Scope of part; limitation.

Sec. 5660. This part does not do the following:

(a) Impair or supersede a legal right a parent, patient, advocate, legal guardian, or other individual may have to consent to or refuse medical treatment on behalf of another.

(b) Create a presumption about a terminally ill patient's desire to receive or refuse medical treatment, regardless of the ability of the patient to participate in medical treatment decisions.

(c) Limit the ability of a court making a determination about a terminally ill patient's medical treatment decisions to take into consideration all of the following state interests:

(i) The preservation of life.

(ii) The prevention of suicide.

(iii) The protection of innocent third parties.

(iv) The preservation of the integrity of the medical profession.

(d) Condone, authorize, or approve suicide, assisted suicide, mercy killing, or euthanasia.

History: Add. 1996, Act 594, Eff. Mar. 31, 1997.

333.5661 Fraud resulting in death of patient; violation as felony; penalty.

Sec. 5661. (1) An individual shall not, by fraud, cause or attempt to cause a patient, patient surrogate, or patient advocate to make a medical treatment decision that results in the death of the patient with the intent to benefit financially from the outcome of the medical treatment decision. As used in this subsection, "fraud" means a false representation of a matter of fact, whether by words or by conduct, by false or misleading allegations, or by concealment of that which should have been disclosed, that deceives and is intended to deceive another so that he or she acts upon it to his or her legal injury.

(2) An individual who violates subsection (1) is guilty of a felony, punishable by imprisonment for not more than 4 years or a fine of not more than $2,000.00, or both.

History: Add. 1996, Act 594, Eff. Mar. 31, 1997.

333.16221 Investigation of licensee, registrant, or applicant for licensure or registration; hearings, oaths, and testimony; report; grounds for proceeding under § 333.16226.

Sec. 16221. The department may investigate activities related to the practice of a health profession by a licensee, a registrant, or an applicant for licensure or registration. The department may hold hearings, administer oaths, and order relevant testimony to be taken and shall report its findings to the appropriate disciplinary subcommittee. The disciplinary subcommittee shall proceed under section 16226 if it finds that 1 or more of the following grounds exist:

(a) A violation of general duty, consisting of negligence or failure to exercise due care, including negligent delegation to or supervision of employees or other individuals, whether or not injury results, or any conduct, practice, or condition which impairs, or may impair, the ability to safely and skillfully practice the health profession.

(b) Personal disqualifications, consisting of 1 or more of the following:

(i) Incompetence.

(ii) Subject to sections 16165 to 16170a, substance abuse as defined in section 6107.

(iii) Mental or physical inability reasonably related to and adversely affecting the licensee's ability to practice in a safe and competent manner.

(iv) Declaration of mental incompetence by a court of competent jurisdiction.

(v) Conviction of a misdemeanor punishable by imprisonment for a maximum term of 2 years; a misdemeanor involving the illegal delivery, possession, or use of a controlled substance; or a felony. A certified copy of the court record is conclusive evidence of the conviction.

(vi) Lack of good moral character.

(vii) Conviction of a criminal offense under sections 520a to 520l of the Michigan penal code, Act No. 328 of the Public Acts of 1931, being sections 750.520a to 750.520l of the Michigan Compiled Laws. A certified copy of the court record is conclusive evidence of the conviction.

(viii) Conviction of a violation of section 492a of the Michigan penal code, Act No. 328 of the Public Acts of 1931, being section 750.492a of the Michigan Compiled Laws. A certified copy of the court record is conclusive evidence of the conviction.

(ix) Conviction of a misdemeanor or felony involving fraud in obtaining or attempting to obtain fees related to the practice of a health profession. A certified copy of the court record is conclusive evidence of the conviction.

(x) Final adverse administrative action by a licensure, registration, disciplinary, or certification board involving the holder of, or an applicant for, a license or registration regulated by another state or a territory of the United States. A certified copy of the record of the board is conclusive evidence of the final action.

(xi) Conviction of a misdemeanor that is reasonably related to or that adversely affects the licensee's ability to practice in a safe and competent manner. A certified copy of the court record is conclusive evidence of the conviction.

(c) Prohibited acts, consisting of 1 or more of the following:

(i) Fraud or deceit in obtaining or renewing a license or registration.

(ii) Permitting the license or registration to be used by an unauthorized person.

(iii) Practice outside the scope of a license.

(iv) Obtaining, possessing, or attempting to obtain or possess a controlled substance as defined in section 7104 or a drug as defined in section 7105 without lawful authority; or selling, prescribing, giving away, or administering drugs for other than lawful diagnostic or therapeutic purposes.

(d) Unethical business practices, consisting of 1 or more of the following:

(i) False or misleading advertising.

(ii) Dividing fees for referral of patients or accepting kickbacks on medical or surgical services, appliances, or medications purchased by or in behalf of patients.

(iii) Fraud or deceit in obtaining or attempting to obtain third party reimbursement.

(e) Unprofessional conduct, consisting of 1 or more of the following:

(i) Misrepresentation to a consumer or patient or in obtaining or attempting to obtain third party reimbursement in the course of professional practice.

(ii) Betrayal of a professional confidence.

(iii) Promotion for personal gain of an unnecessary drug, device, treatment, procedure, or service.

(iv) Directing or requiring an individual to purchase or secure a drug, device, treatment, procedure, or service from another person, place, facility, or business in which the licensee has a financial interest.

(f) Failure to report a change of name or mailing address within 30 days after the change occurs.

(g) A violation, or aiding or abetting in a violation, of this article or of a rule promulgated under this article.

(h) Failure to comply with a subpoena issued pursuant to this part, failure to respond to a complaint issued under this article or article 7, failure to appear at a compliance or an administrative hearing, or failure to report under section 16222 or 16223.

(i) Failure to pay an installment of an assessment levied pursuant to section 2504 of the insurance code of 1956, Act No. 218 of the Public Acts of 1956, being section 500.2504 of the Michigan Compiled Laws, within 60 days after notice by the appropriate board.

(j) A violation of section 17013 or 17513.

(k) Failure to meet 1 or more of the requirements for licensure or registration under section 16174.

(l) A violation of section 17015 or 17515.

(m) A violation of section 17016 or 17516.

(n) A violation of section 5654 or 5655.

History: 1978, Act 368, Eff. Sept. 30, 1978;—Am. 1986, Act 174, Imd. Eff. July 7, 1986;—Am. 1986, Act 195, Imd. Eff. July 8, 1986;—Am. 1986, Act 319, Imd. Eff. Dec. 26, 1986;—Am. 1987, Act 178, Imd. Eff. Nov. 19, 1987;—Am. 1989, Act 15, Imd. Eff. May 15, 1989;—Am. 1993, Act 79, Eff. Apr. 1, 1994;—Am. 1993, Act 133, Eff. Apr. 1, 1994;—Am. 1995, Act 196, Imd. Eff. Nov. 22, 1995;—Am. 1996, Act 273, Eff. Mar. 31, 1997;—Am. 1996, Act 540, Imd. Eff. Jan. 15, 1997;—Am. 1996, Act 594, Eff. Mar. 31, 1997.

Compiler's note: Section 3 of Act 174 of 1986 provides: "This amendatory act shall only apply to contested cases filed on or after July 1, 1986."

Compiler's note: Section 2 of Act 319 of 1986 provides: "Section 16221(e)(iv) of Act No. 368 of the Public Acts of 1978, as added by this amendatory act, shall take effect April 1, 1987."

Compiler's note: Subdivision "(n)" evidently should be designated as subdivision "(o)" and subdivision (n) should read as follows: "(n) Failure to comply with section 9206(3)."

333.16226 Sanctions; determination; judicial review; maximum fine for violation of § 333.16221(a) or (b); completion of program or examination.

Sec. 16226. (1) After finding the existence of 1 or more of the grounds for disciplinary subcommittee action listed in section 16221, a disciplinary subcommittee shall impose 1 or more of the following sanctions for each violation:

Violations of Section 16221	Sanctions
Subdivision(a), (b)(ii), (b)(iv), (b)(vi), or (b)(vii)	Probation, limitation, denial, suspension, revocation, restitution, community service, or fine.
Subdivision (b)(viii)	Revocation or denial.

Subdivision (b)(i), (b)(iii), (b)(v), (b)(ix), (b)(x), or (b)(xi)	Limitation, suspension, revocation, denial, probation, restitution, community service, or fine.
Subdivision (c)(i)	Denial, revocation, suspension, probation, limitation, community service, or fine.
Subdivision (c)(ii)	Denial, suspension, revocation, restitution, community service, or fine.
Subdivision (c)(iii)	Probation, denial, suspension, revocation, restitution, community service, or fine.
Subdivision (c)(iv) or (d)(iii)	Fine, probation, denial, suspension, revocation, community service, or restitution.
Subdivision (d)(i) or (d)(ii)	Reprimand, fine, probation, community service, denial, or restitution.
Subdivision (e)(i)	Reprimand, fine, probation, limitation, suspension, community service, denial, or restitution.
Subdivision (e)(ii) or (h)	Reprimand, probation, suspension, restitution, community service, denial, or fine.
Subdivision (e)(iii) or (e)(iv)	Reprimand, fine, probation, suspension, revocation, limitation, community service, denial, or restitution.
Subdivision (f)	Reprimand or fine.
Subdivision (g)	Reprimand, probation, denial, suspension, revocation, limitation, restitution, community service, or fine.
Subdivision (i)	Suspension or fine.
Subdivision (j) or (n)	Reprimand or fine.
Subdivision (k)	Reprimand, denial, or limitation.
Subdivision (l)	Denial, revocation, restitution, probation, suspension, limitation, reprimand, or fine.
Subdivision (m)	Revocation or denial.

(2) Determination of sanctions for violations under this section shall be made by a disciplinary subcommittee. If, during judicial review, the court of appeals determines that a final decision or order of a disciplinary subcommittee prejudices substantial rights of the petitioner for 1 or more of the grounds listed in section 106 of the administrative procedures act of 1969, being section 24.306 of Michigan Compiled Laws, and holds that the final decision order is unlawful and is to be set aside, the court shall state on the

record the reasons for the holding and may remand the case to the disciplinary subcommittee for further consideration.

(3) A disciplinary subcommittee may impose a fine of up to, but not exceeding, $250,000.00 for a violation of section 16221(a) or (b).

(4) A disciplinary subcommittee may require a licensee or registrant or an applicant for licensure or registration who has violated this article or article 7 or a rule promulgated under this article or article 7 to satisfactorily complete an education program, a training program, or a treatment program, a mental, physical, or professional competence examination, or a combination of those programs and examinations.

History: 1978, Act 368, Eff. Sept. 30, 1978;—Am. 1986, Act 174, Imd. Eff. July 7, 1986;—Am. 1986, Act 195, Imd. Eff. July 8, 1986;—Am. 1986, Act, 319, Imd. Eff. Dec. 26, 1986;—Am. 1987, Act 178, Imd. Eff. Nov. 19, 1987;—Am. 1989, Act 15, Imd. Eff. May 15, 1989;—Am. 1993, Act 79, Eff. Apr. 1, 1994;—Am. 1993, Act 133. Eff. Apr. 1, 1994;—Am. 1996, Act 273, Eff. Mar. 31, 1997;—Am. 1996, Act 540, Imd. Eff. Jan. 15, 1997;—Am. 1996, Act 594, Eff. Mar. 31, 1997.

Compiler's note: Section 3 of Act 174 of 1986 provides: "This amendatory act shall only apply to contested cases filed on or after July 1, 1986."

Compiler's note: In subsection (1), "Subdivision (j) or (n)" evidently should read "Subdivision (j) or (o)" and "Subdivision (l)" evidently should read "Subdivision (l) or (n)." See Compiler's note to § 333.16221.

Glossary

Active Dying The time before death when the body begins to break down. Various bodily functions cease, and the resulting complications become impossible to control. The process can last as long as two months but often takes only a few days.

Adverse Drug Reaction An unintended and negative side effect of a drug, varying from very mild to severe. It can threaten a person's life.

Aggressive Medical Treatment The use of high-tech medical and pharmacological interventions in treating a serious medical condition. The goal is to cure or to minimize morbidity. **High-tech medicine** can also be used for palliation of symptoms and pain in terminal illness.

Agitation The condition of a person who is extremely fitful, restless, and anxious. Agitation can result from a number of causes: extreme physical discomfort, brain tumors, **cognitive impairment**, metabolic disturbances, **constipation**, drug interactions, or toxicities.

Anal Catheter See **Rectal Tube.**

Antibiotic A class of drugs used to fight bacterial infections.

Area Agencies on Aging Created by the Older Americans Act, these agencies support and monitor programs for the elderly at the local level.

Attending Physician The staff physician who supervises the training and work of physicians-in-training. The attending physician has ultimate responsibility for patient care.

Bedsore See **Decubitus Ulcer.**

Brain Metastases   Malignant tumors that have migrated to the brain from a primary cancer site.

"Braty" Diet   Diet restricted to *b*ananas, *r*ice, *a*pple juice, *t*oast (dry), and *y*ogurt which is used to control diarrhea.

Breakthrough Pain   Pain that is not controlled by the normal amount of pain medication.

Cardiopulmonary Resuscitation (CPR)   A technique for restarting the heart and lungs after they have stopped functioning. This is routinely used in hospitals when a patient suffers a cardiac arrest.

Caregiver   The person who assumes primary responsibility for delivering care. Often several people share in this task, in which case it is usually carried out in serial fashion, so that at any one time, only one person is responsible.

Care Plan   The organization of care for a patient. It involves all the necessary medical, nursing, and therapeutic interventions, as well as the scheduling of people who will help carry out the plan.

Case Manager   A case manager is usually a nurse practitioner who is assigned to help facilitate the management of the patient's hospital stay. This person is also responsible for making sure that the patient is discharged as soon as medically feasible.

Catheterization   The insertion of a tube into the urethra to empty the bladder. This can be done intermittently on an as-needed basis, or permanently by means of a catheter inserted by a nurse.

Chemotherapy   Any pharmaceutical treatment for disease. It is frequently used for cancer.

Cheyne-Stokes   An intermittent, irregular breathing pattern that often precedes death. It may be seen in certain cardiac and neurological diseases.

Chief of Service   The physician in charge of a specific division in a hospital, such as internal medicine.

Cognitive Impairment   Impairment of mental capabilities, which can occur in varying degrees.

Coma Complete loss of any sensory awareness. In this uncon-scious state only the basic brain-stem functions operate. A person in a coma requires intravenous nutrition and hydration to survive.

Commode A bedside toilet.

Condom Catheter A condom catheter for urine incontinence; can be fitted over a man's penis. Also called a **Texas catheter.**

Constipation A condition in which the feces are hardened and bowel movements are difficult and infrequent. It can result from lack of exercise, inadequate diet, or dehydration or be the side effect of a medication.

Continuity of Care The practice of having a team or individual responsible for making sure that one **care plan** is followed and that those involved in the caregiving adhere to it. Continuity of care also implies that the same people or group of people will work with the patient, and that service will be available when needed.

Continuous Care When a hospice patient's symptoms cannot be managed or when the caregiver is incapacitated, it is possible to receive twenty-four-hour in-home care from hospice. This care usu-ally lasts no more than seventy-two hours, but in extreme cases can last for four days.

Decubitus Ulcer A sore that results from unrelieved pressure on the skin. It is caused by debility, lack of exercise, inadequate nutri-tion, **incontinence,** and prolonged bed rest. It first appears as a red spot, typically in a place where the bone and skin are in contact. It can be controlled by frequent turning, ensuring moderate exercise, gentle rubbing of the affected spot, and relieving pressure on the area.

Discharge Planner The person on the hospital staff, usually a nurse or social worker, who is responsible for planning the patient's discharge from the hospital. The discharge planner can help the family arrange for home care or an institutional placement.

Disimpaction The process of manually removing impacted feces from the bowel. Only someone trained in this procedure should attempt it.

Do Not Resuscitate (DNR)   A physician's order that means that if a patient has a cardiac arrest or respiration ceases, no attempt should be made to intervene to save the person's life. The person should be allowed to die.

Durable Medical Equipment (DME)   Equipment used in the care of a sick person at home, such as a hospital bed, commode, or walker. It can be rented or purchased from a DME company or sometimes borrowed from the "loan closet" of the agency caring for the dying person.

Durable Power of Attorney   A durable power of attorney refers to a document in which a competent adult assigns specific decision-making rights to a specified person who must be at least eighteen years old. In a **Durable Medical Power of Attorney** one adult assigns another person the right to make decisions pertaining to the assigning person's medical care. A **Durable Financial Power of Attorney** gives another person the right to make specified financial decisions and to sign specified financial documents such as checks on a mortgage. Both of these come into effect after two physicians certify that the person who assigned the power of attorney is no longer capable of understanding or communicating.

Egg Crate Mattress   A foam rubber mattress whose shape resembles an egg crate. It is used to prevent bedsores.

Electrocardiogram   A measurement of heart rhythms by means of electrodes taped to various places on the body.

Emergency Medical Service (EMS)   The personnel who staff an ambulance. An EMT is an emergency medical technician.

Enema   Injection of a liquid into the colon via the anus for the purposes of emptying the bowel.

Enterostomal Therapist   A therapist specifically trained to manage ostomies and wound care. ETs work for hospitals and **durable medical equipment** companies and can be used as consultants in the care of a bedsore. Nurses can also provide wound care.

External Catheter   A type of **venous access device** which can be directly connected to **intravenous** tubing.

Family Rounds A time during the day when all the people participating in caregiving who are available sit down and discuss the problems and issues involved in their task.

Fellow A physician receiving postresidency training.

Foley Catheter A catheter inserted by a trained professional directly into the bladder. It remains there, allowing the bladder to drain freely into a Foley bag.

Gurney A trolley bed used to transport patients around the hospital. It is sometimes used to move a person in and out of an ambulance.

Hallucinations The perception of sights or sounds that are not actually present. Drug reactions and diseases that affect brain functioning can cause hallucinations.

Health Maintenance Organization (HMO) A prepaid health insurance plan. Clinic visits are free or very inexpensive. Physicians control the patient's access to more costly forms of care.

Heroic Measures The use of **cardiopulmonary resuscitation,** technological interventions such as a mechanical **ventilator,** or pharmacological interventions such as **antibiotics** to prolong life.

High-tech Medicine Machines used in treating and diagnosing disease.

Home (Health) Care Agency An agency that provides both chronic long-term care for homebound patients and care for recently discharged patients. Although some have a subsidiary that offers hospice care, home care agencies as such are not licensed to provide Medicare-reimbursable **hospice** care.

Home Health Aide A person trained to assist the patient in washing, dressing, eating, and transfers.

Hospice A philosophy of care. In the Medicare reimbursement system, which is copied by most private insurers, the hospice benefit can be activated when a physician certifies that a person is likely to have only six months left to live. The benefit provides hours of **home health aide** care a week and regular nursing visits. Physician visits to the home, medications, and the rental of **durable medical equipment** are also covered. Other special services such as physical therapy and social work may be covered. Hospice programs include spiritual counseling and support for the family. They also rely on the involvement of trained volunteers.

House Officer   A name for a **resident** or **intern.**

Incontinence   The spontaneous uncontrolled expulsion of the contents of the bladder or bowel.

In-Dwelling Catheter   See **Venous Access Device.**

Infusion Pump   A device that provides medication directly into the patient's body by means of either a **subcutaneous** catheter or an **intrathecal** or **intravenous** device. On some pumps the patient may control the amount of pain medication received.

Instrumental Support   Practical support for the caregiver and those providing hands-on care. Examples are: shopping, child care, managing bills and insurance, and house maintenance. The types of instrumental support are limitless.

Intern   A medical school graduate taking an additional year of training before becoming a licensed physician.

Intrathecal   Into the spinal canal.

Intravenous (IV)   Within the vein. Medication, nutrition, and hydration can be supplied intravenously. An **infusion pump** is used to administer this form of therapy. In many cases, it is now possible to have IV therapy at home.

Intravenous Hydration   The process of giving fluid intravenously to someone who is unable to swallow liquids.

Life Support Systems   High-tech machines in intensive care units which keep extremely ill people alive.

Living Will   A statement, signed by the person making it, specifying in advance that no **heroic measures** be taken to prolong his or her life. The U.S. Supreme Court has ruled that such a statement is legally binding on the hospital if it is drawn up according to the specific state laws.

Medicaid   The government health insurance coverage available to the poor. Eligibility and benefits are determined by individual states.

Medical Rounds   Teaching sessions in which **attending physicians** discuss specific patients with **medical students** or **interns** either in the patient's room or in the hall.

Medical Student   Physician in training. Four years of medical school and one year of advanced training are the minimum education requirements for becoming licensed as a physician.

Medicare   The basic government-funded insurance available to most people over sixty-five. It includes a **hospice** benefit.

Nursing Home   A facility typically used for long-term chronic care. If the family cannot care for a dying person, the patient may be admitted to a nursing home. Most nursing homes cannot care for patients who require significant amounts of nursing or skilled care. Also called a skilled nursing facility.

Nutritional Supplement   Commonly used by cancer patients who have trouble eating. There are many such products on the market. A dietitian can provide information about which supplement would be appropriate for the dying person's needs.

Ombudsman's Office for Aging Affairs   The office that, in most states, deals with affairs of the aging. If it becomes necessary to institutionalize a dying patient, this office can be consulted for information on available nursing homes.

Out-of-Pocket   Those costs not covered by insurance and which the caregiver and/or dying person must pay for.

Palliative Care   Care limited to controlling pain and managing the symptoms of a terminal illness. It is not intended to prolong the patient's life. In reality this distinction is sometimes difficult to make.

Patient Log   A record kept by the caregiver of when medication is given, the dose, the response of the person, and any significant observations the caregiver wishes to make.

Perineal Care   Care of the perineum, the area of the anus and genitals.

Peripheral Intravenous Catheter (PIC Line)   A type of **venous access device** for administering medication directly into a vein. It can be inserted in the home and remain in place for up to six months.

Phased Discharge   Discharge to a lower level of care before the patient returns home.

Port   A type of **venous access device** inserted under the skin which allows medication to be injected directly into a vein with little or no discomfort to the patient.

Posey Jacket   A loose-fitting vest used to secure the patient to the bed while allowing freedom of movement for the arms.

Pro Re Nata (PRN)   On an as-needed basis.

Prospective Payment System   The **Medicare** reimbursement system for hospitals. Hospitals are paid a set rate for each diagnosis-related group regardless of the hospital's actual costs.

"Pulling the Plug"   A slang term for turning off life support systems.

Rectal Tube   A bag that fits snugly around the anus and sticks to the skin. It can be drained every three to five days depending on the consistency of the feces and leakage. It minimizes skin irritation from diarrhea.

Resident   See **Intern.**

Respite   A technical term meaning a break from caregiving. The **hospice** benefit recognizes the need for respite by allowing hospice patients to be hospitalized for up to five days a month to give the caregiver a rest.

Seizure   An uncontrolled electrical firing in the brain. It affects cognition and/or behavior and may cause convulsions.

Skin Patch   A skin patch is a method for delivering medication directly into the body via the skin.

Subcutaneous   Beneath the skin.

Sublingual   Under the tongue. Sublingual is a route for delivering pain medication.

Suctioning   A process by which a tube is inserted through a patient's mouth and down the throat to remove fluids from the airways.

Texas Catheter   See **Condom Catheter.**

Transfer   The technique of moving a person from the bed to a chair, commode, gurney, or other place. Caregivers should be trained by a professional to perform transfers. This will reduce the danger of injury to the caregiver or patient.

Universal Precautions   Simple measures to prevent the spread of a disease (such as HIV) from patient to caregiver.

Urinal   A hand-held receptacle used for urinating in bed. There are separate types of urinals designed for men and women.

Venous Access Device   A device that allows repeated access to a vein through an opening made in the skin. It may take the form of a **peripheral intravenous catheter,** which may be inserted in the home by a qualified professional, or an **external catheter** or an implanted **port,** both of which must be inserted by a doctor in a hospital or out-patient setting.

Ventilator   A machine that takes over the breathing functions, via a tube inserted into the trachea, for someone unable to breathe on his or her own.

Walker   A four-legged device that assists people in retaining their balance and therefore helps them to walk on their own.

Bibliography

Asheervath, J., and D. Blevins. 1986. *The Handbook of Clinical Nursing Practice.* Norwalk, CT: Appleton-Century-Crofts.

Bartlett, J., and A. K. Finkbeiner. 1998. *The Guide to Living with HIV Infection,* 4th edition. Baltimore: Johns Hopkins University Press.

Biglow-Kemp, B., and A. Pillitteri. 1984. *Fundamentals of Nursing: A Framework for Practice.* Boston: Little, Brown.

Burnell, G. 1993. *Final Choices: To Live or to Die in an Age of Medical Technology.* New York: Plenum Publishing, Insight Books.

Claiborn, R. 1982. "A Patient Looks at Pain and Analgesia." *Hospital Practice* 17 (9): 24–33.

Coons, D., L. Metzelaar, A. Robinson, and B. Spencer. 1986. *A Better Life.* Columbus, OH: Source for Nursing Home Literature.

Dalton, W. S. 1985. "Rational Use of Narcotic Analgesics." *Hospital Therapy,* September, 45–60.

DiGregorio, G. J., et al. 1991. *Handbook of Pain Management,* 3rd edition. West Chester, PA: Medical Surveillance.

Foley, K. 1985. "The Treatment of Cancer Pain." *New England Journal of Medicine* 313 (2): 84–95.

Frankenhauser, M. P., and S. B. Shanfield. 1985. "When—and When Not—to Use Psychotropic Drugs." *Hospital Therapy,* October, 43–52.

Harwell, A. 1995. *Ready to Live: Prepare to Die.* Wheaton, IL: Harold Shaw.

Kennedy, P. H. 1982. *Dying at Home with Cancer.* Springfield, IL: Charles C. Thomas.

Kessler, D. 1997. *The Rights of the Dying.* New York: Harper.

Kilburn, Linda H. 1988. *The Hospice Operations Manual.* Arlington, VA: National Hospice Organization.

Lattanzi-Licht, M., J. Mahoney, and G. Miller. 1998. *The Hospice Choice.* New York: Simon & Schuster.

Lerner, G. 1985. *A Death of One's Own.* Madison: University of Wisconsin Press.

Mace, N. L., and P. V. Rabins. 1999. *The 36-Hour Day*, 3rd edition. Baltimore: Johns Hopkins University Press.

Marks, R. M., and E. J. Sachar. 1973. "Undertreatment of Medical In-Patients with Narcotic Analgesics." *Annals of Internal Medicine* 76 (2): 173–81.

Meinhart, N. T., and M. McCaffery. 1983. *Pain: A Nursing Approach to Assessment and Analysis.* New York: Appleton-Century-Crofts.

Melzack, R. 1990. "The Tragedy of Needless Pain." *Scientific American* 262 (2): 27–33.

Mor, V., D. S. Greer, and R. Kastenbaum. 1988. *The Hospice Experiment.* Report of the National Hospice Study. Baltimore: Johns Hopkins University Press.

Moulin, D. E., and K. M. Foley. 1984. "Management of Pain in Patients with Cancer." *Psychiatric Annals* 14 (11): 815–22.

Newshar, G. T., and S. F. Wainapel. 1993. "Pain Characteristics and Their Management in Persons with AIDS." *JANAC* 4 (2): 53–59.

Pitel, M., and M. Wemett. 1964. "The Injection." *American Journal of Nursing* 64 (4): 101–11.

Plezia, P., and D. S. Alberts. 1985. "Integrated Approach to Cancer Pain Treatment." *Hospital Therapy,* September, 20–25.

Plezia, P., and J. Linford. 1985. "Innovative Approaches to Refractory Pain." *Hospital Therapy,* October, 25–42.

Reuler, J. B., D. E. Dirard, and D. A. Nardone. 1980. "The Chronic Pain Syndrome: Misconceptions and Management." *Annals of Internal Medicine* 93: 588–96.

Timby, B. K. 1989. *Clinical Nursing Procedures*. Philadelphia: Lippincott.

Wallis, L., R. M. Galvin, and D. Thompson. 1984. "Unlocking Pain's Secrets." *Time* 123 (24): 58–66.

Zerwekh, J. V. 1983. "The Dehydration Question." *Nursing 83* 13 (1): 47–51.

Index

Names appearing in boldface designate those who died.

A

Acquired immune deficiency syndrome. *See* AIDS.

Active dying, 12, 180–81, 209

Adverse drug reactions, 8, 29, 213–18, 232, 235

Agitation, 6, 8, 61, 74, 225–26

Aides. *See* Home health aides.

AIDS (acquired immune deficiency syndrome). *See also* Smith, Joyce.
  and caregiving, 250–60
  end-of-life decisions, 259–60
  fear of, xx, 120–21, 184, 251
  home care needs, 254–57
  infection precautions, 254–56
  and infectious wastes, 37, 218, 254–56
  and Medicaid, 65
  pain, 257–58
  patient rights, 258–60
  physician, 54
  support groups, 251
  symptoms of, 32, 170, 253

Alternative therapies. *See also* Exercise; Massage; Music; Nutrition; Spiritual support.
  laughter, 144–45
  marijuana, 211, 214
  relaxation, 223, 235–36
  visualization, 236–37
  yoga, 131, 241

Alzheimer's disease. *See* Roehm, Carl.

American Cancer Society, 30, 238

American Pain Society, 238–39

Amyotrophic lateral sclerosis (ALS), xix

Anal catheter, 217

Anger, 6, 134–36

Antiretroviral therapy, 251

Appetite, 8, 213

Area agencies on aging, 26, 242

Assets, transfer of. *See* Will, preparation of.

Autonomy, 2, 9, 47, 110, 198. *See also* Ethical dilemmas, medication, cessation of.

B

Bathing, 49, 72, 175, 202–3, 236

Bed, patient, 30–34. *See also* Transfers; Turning.

Bedsore. *See* Decubitus ulcer.

Benefits, survivors', 195–97

Bereavement counseling, 55, 149, 243. *See also* Grief.

Bowel, ruptured, 45

Brain cancer. *See* Jim DeMott; Elizabeth Krolick.

"Braty" diet, 217
Breakthrough pain, 230
Breast cancer. *See* Elizabeth Krolick.
Breathing, 35, 154, 230
  Cheyne-Stokes, 137, 154
  near-death, 161–62, 164, 166, 168, 174

C
Cancer
  American Cancer Society, 30, 238
  bone, 37, 231
  brain (*see* Jim DeMott; Elizabeth Krolick)
  breast (*see* Elizabeth Krolick)
  Department of Public Health, 78, 238
  leukemia (*see* Lisa Knott)
  liver (*see* Herbert Wolf; John Wright)
  lung (*see* Anthony Lane; Lawrence Quinn; Dorothy Stead)
  Oncology Nurses Association, 232, 238
  ovarian (*see* Alice Clark)
  testicular (*see* John Wright)
Cancer hotline, 231
Cardiopulmonary resuscitation (CPR), 40, 155
Care partner, 3
Care plan, 26–27, 50, 65–66
Caregiver
  care plan, 26–27, 50, 65–66
  daily routine of, 51–52, 80, 125–28
  deciding to become, 1, 6, 11–13, 40–41, 52, 67–68, 99–100, 106, 149–51
  definition of, 2
  developing daily routine for, 125–28, 133
  emotions of, 118, 131, 138. *See also* Death, actual, fear of; Grief.
  evaluation of, 130–31
  hospital role of, 17–25, 29–30
  household tasks, managing, 51–52 (*see also* Informal support)
  numerous decisions of, 127
  physical and emotional strains on, 5, 10, 12, 37–38, 77, 128–32
  proper training and, 220
  satisfactions of, 1, 6, 79, 99
  setting limits and, 145–46
  stamina of, 5, 13, 50–52
Caregiving, hands-on, 20–21, 29–30, 62, 105–6, 201. *See also* Alternative therapies; Bathing; Decubitus ulcer (bedsore); Catheterization; Disimpaction; Elimination; Exercise; Feeding, patient; Hygiene; Medication; Mouth care; Suctioning; Transfers.
  disimpaction, 30, 45, 162, 218
  enema, 30, 85
  eye care, 222
  genitalia, care of, 11, 150, 203
  grooming, 202
  hair care, 202
  injections, 31, 43, 227–29
  massage, 167, 204, 224, 235
  nail care, 202
  nausea, 209, 211, 213–14
  turning, 37, 202, 204–7
  wound dressing, 44, 82, 204
Case manager, 59
Catheterization, 30, 84–85, 216–17, 226. *See also* Elimination.
  Foley catheter, 84, 216–17
  Texas catheter, 216

Cheyne-Stokes breathing, 137, 154. *See also* Breathing, near-death.

Children
  and AIDS, 254
  and caregiver, 51, 110, 140
  dying (*see* Lisa Knott; David Steiner)
  and the dying, 99, 115–18, 145, 173–74, 180
  and viewing the body. *See* Death, after, and children.

Clark, Alice, xvii, 16, 105, 159–61

Clark, Stan (caregiver), 16, 33–34, 39, 50, 61, 80–81, 92–93, 102, 107, 113, 127, 146, 147, 150, 159–61, 188–89, 209, 215, 235, 236

Code status, 23, 38

Cognitive impairment, 7, 18, 23, 224, 253. *See also* Hallucination.
  definition of, 83, 224–25

Coma, 37, 138

Condoms, 216

Constipation, 8, 174, 216, 217–18, 235

Continuous care, 42–43

Costs, out-of-pocket, 50–51, 65

CPR (cardiopulmonary resuscitation), 40

D
Death, actual
  caregiver accounts of, 152–53, 158–80
  confirmation of, 137–38
  description of, 12, 137–38, 152–54
  fear of, 12, 136–38, 149, 152–53, 160–61, 163–64
  hospital rates of, 19–20

media portrayal of, 45, 152–53
pronouncement of, 155–56

Death, after. *See also* Grief.
  and children, 156–57, 163, 168, 174, 177, 180, 185
  death benefits, 195–97
  death certificate, 155, 161, 195–96, 249
  donation of body, 180
  funeral, 46, 155, 182–87
  practical matters, 195–97
  removal of body, 156, 162–63, 179–80
  will, preparation of, 194–95

Death, impending. *See also* Active dying.
  vs. acute, reversible condition, 36
  caregiver preparation for, 45, 136–38
  denial of, 24, 47–48, 79, 121, 131–32, 135
  and hospice, 46, 53
  hospitalization for, 38–40
  informing patient of, 24, 63
  patient preparation for, 24, 46, 134
  prediction of, 8, 72–73, 85, 133–34, 137
  signs of, 5, 72, 84, 85–86, 136–38, 153–54. *See also* Breathing, near-death; Death, actual, caregiver accounts of.

Death benefits, 195–97

Death certificate, 155, 161, 195–96, 248

Decadron (dexamethasone), 28, 83

Decubitus ulcer (bedsore), xx, 23, 150, 203–7. *See also* Bathing.

Dementia. *See* Cognitive impairment.

DeMott, Jim, xvii, 16, 161–63, 218

DeMott, Lucille (caregiver), 16,
    18–21, 23–24, 28, 34–35, 44, 49,
    52, 56, 61, 62, 71–72, 73, 74, 75,
    77–78, 81, 84, 90–91, 92, 98,
    102, 105, 111, 116–17, 122–23,
    129, 146, 161–63, 183–84
Department of Public Health, 78,
    238
Depression, 12. *See also* Suicide.
Diarrhea, 95, 215–17
Diet. *See* Nutrition.
Dignity, 1, 11, 18, 92–94, 105, 202.
    See also Autonomy.
Discharge, hospital, 25–35, 65–66
Discharge planner, 14, 26, 30–35,
    65–69
Disimpaction, 30, 45, 162, 218
DME. *See* Durable medical
    equipment.
DNR (Do not resuscitate), 155–56,
    248
Drinking, patient, 208–12, 218
Drugs. *See* Medication.
Durable medical equipment
    (DME), 31–32, 33–34, 203, 220
Durable power of attorney, 240,
    260–61
Dying, active, 12, 180–81, 209

E
Elimination
    commode for, 31
    and control loss, 160, 215–18,
        225
    unaided, importance of, 32
Emergency medical service
    (EMS), 154–56, 169
Enema, 30, 85
Equipment technicians, 31. *See
    also* Durable medical
    equipment.
Ethical dilemmas
    comfort vs. treatment, 83–87,

162. *See also* Pain control;
    Quality of life.
medication, cessation of, 23–24,
    83–87. *See also* Autonomy;
    Intravenous (IV) hydration.
use of life support, 4, 40–41, 83–
    87. *See also* DNR; Life
    support systems; Living will.
Exercise
    and appetite, 213
    and bedsores, 203–4
    isometric, 223, 236
    and sleep, 223, 224
External catheter, 229. *See also*
    Catheterization.
Eye care, 222

F
Family, 2, 36, 87–92, 102–3. *See also*
    Children; Informal support.
Family rounds, 91, 92
Feeding, of patient. *See also*
    Mouth care.
    appetite, 8, 213
    forced, warning against, 154,
        213
    in hospital, 21, 30
    tricks to, 30, 212–13
Fever, 36
Foley catheter, 84, 216–17
Formal support
    agencies, 53–59. *See also* Health
        maintenance organization;
        Home health care agency;
        Hospice.
    caregiver's employer as, 51
    functions of, 42–47, 100
    groups, 51, 143–44
    insurance for, 42–43, 69, 75. *See
        also* Insurance; Medicare.
    obtaining, 65–69. *See also*
        Discharge, hospital; Discharge
        planner.

problems with, 47–48, 62, 76–78, 81–82
professionals, 59–64. *See also* Home health aides; Nurses; Physicians; Professionals, types of.
selection of, 69–71, 73–76
Friends. *See* Informal support.
Funeral, 46, 156, 182–87

G
Genitalia care, 11, 150, 203
Grief. *See also* Bereavement counseling.
anticipatory, 131–32
personal accounts of, 188–94
therapy, 143–44, 242–44
Grooming, 202. *See also* Hygiene.

H
Hair care, 202. *See also* Hygiene.
Hallucination, 74, 116, 135, 154, 224–25
Health maintenance organization (HMO), 58–59, 70, 75
Hemlock Soceity, 158, 242. *See also* Suicide.
Heroic measure, 38, 40, 155. *See also* Ethical dilemmas, use of life support.
HIV. *See* AIDS.
HMO. *See* Health maintenance organization.
Home death, 198–200
reasons against, 39
reasons for, 47, 94, 156
trend to, 1–5
Home health aides. *See also* Formal support.
duties of, 10–11, 42, 56, 56n, 63–64
friendships with, 50, 64

reimbursement for, 10, 64
selection of, 69–71, 73–76
supervision of, 71–73
Home health care agency vs. hospice, 53–59
physicians and, 34, 58–60, 64, 68–69, 247–48
selection of, 65–71
Hospice. *See also* Bereavement counseling
in-patient, 5, 38, 42, 53
philosophy, 4, 53–57, 91
physicians, 48, 53–54, 62, 247–48
vs. home care, 58
Hospitalization
caregiver role in, 17–25, 29–30
of the dying, 5, 20, 38–39, 65
for pain control, 5, 26, 37, 82
for respite, 5, 37, 42–43, 52, 148
at teaching hospital, 21–23
Hygiene. *See also* Decubitus ulcer; Elimination.
bathing, 49, 72, 175, 202–3, 236–37
eye care, 222
genitalia care, 11, 150, 203
grooming, 202
hair care, 202
mouth care, 27–28, 30, 154, 167, 210, 212, 214–15. *See also* Nutrition; Swallowing.
nail care, 202
odors, patient, 32

I
In-dwelling catheter. *See* Foley catheter.
Incontinence, 11, 20, 154, 160, 202, 203, 215–17
Informal support
AIDS and, 250–51
children as, 115–18

Informal support *(cont.)*
friends and family as, 11, 36,
102–15, 142–43, 161
lack of, 120–24
organization of, 113–15
problems with, 87–92, 118–20
Infusion pump, 31, 229–30, 234
Injections, 31, 44, 227–29. *See also*
Medication.
Insomnia. *See* Sleep.
Insurance. *See also* Health
maintenance organization;
Medicare.
for caregiver training, 30
home care, 10–11, 42–43, 58, 67,
69, 70
hospice, 11, 42, 53, 54, 54n, 57,
69, 70
life, 196–97
for medical equipment, 32
Intravenous (IV) hydration, 40, 80,
83, 85–86
Intravenous (IV) therapy, 9, 20–21,
229–30, 235
Isometrics, 223, 236. *See also*
Exercise.
IV. *See* Intravenous (IV)
hydration; Intravenous (IV)
therapy.

K
Klein, Lucinda (caregiver), 15, 16,
33, 57, 65, 76–77, 120–21, 134,
135, 136, 141, 144, 150, 151,
170–72. *See also* Smith, Joyce.
Knott, Lisa, xvii–xviii, 16, 164–65
Knott, Pat (caregiver), 16, 43, 44,
48, 73–74, 76, 95, 103, 108, 109,
110–11, 112–13, 119, 141, 142,
143, 147, 148, 149, 164–65, 187,
193–94
Krolick, Anna (caregiver), 16, 24,
26–28, 31, 35, 47, 61, 64, 66, 67,
74, 76, 84–85, 87, 99, 104,
106–7, 109, 111, 112, 113–14,
116, 117, 132, 135, 145, 146,
165–68, 210
Krolick, Elizabeth, xviii, 16, 101,
145, 165–68, 218

L
Lab technicians, 64
Lane, Anthony, xviii–xix, 16. *See
also* Sweet, Laura (caregiver).
Laughter, 144–45
Lazarus syndrome, 251
Leukemia. *See* Lisa Knott.
Life support systems, 38, 40–41,
155–56. *See also* Ethical
dilemmas, use of life support.
Liver cancer. *See* Herbert Wolf;
John Wright.
Living will, 84, 240
Lou Gehrig's disease, xix
Lung cancer. *See* Anthony Lane;
Lawrence Quinn; Dorothy
Stead.

M
Malnutrition, 7. *See also* Nutrition.
Marijuana, 211, 214
Marinol, 211
Marriage, strains on, 140
Martin, Al, xix, 16, 168–69
Martin, Florence (caregiver), 16,
47–48, 49–50, 105, 114, 123,
130, 131, 134, 136, 143, 151,
168–69, 185–86
Massage, 167, 204, 223, 235
Medicaid, 42, 57
Medical equipment. *See* Durable
medical equipment.
Medicare coverage. *See also*
Insurance.
for HMOs, 58–59
for home care, 58

for hospice, 36, 42, 43, 53, 54n, 57
prospective payment system and, 5
Medication
alternate forms of, 19, 28, 29, 226–27
anger and, 136
costs of, 58
intravenous therapy, 9, 20–21, 229–30, 235
monitoring of, 17–18, 35, 82, 86 (*see also* Patient log)
prioritizing, 27
refusal to take, 27–28, 83
scheduling, 29, 81, 86–87
side effects (*see* Adverse drug reactions)
skin patch, 229
sublingual, 229
swallowing of, 27–28, 29
Melzack, R., 88, 232, 245
Memory loss. *See* Cognitive impairment.
Mobility, 81, 218–20
Mor, V., 131
Mouth care, 27–28, 30, 154, 167, 210, 212, 214–15. *See also* Nutrition; Swallowing difficulties.
Music, 46, 99, 105, 116, 179, 183–84, 237

N
Narcotic analgesics
addiction to, 232
Dilaudid, 82, 165, 246
list of, 245–47
morphine, 82, 162, 234–35, 245
physicians and, 82
side effects of, 85
Nausea, 209, 211, 213–14

Nurses. *See also* Formal support.
as discharge planners, 65
home care role of, 43–44, 62–63, 86
hospice vs. home care, 56–57, 155
in hospital, 19–21, 23–24, 29–30, 34
reimbursement for, 30, 57
selection of, 70, 73–76
as teachers to caregiver, 29–30, 43–44, 62, 201
types of, 56n
Nursing home, 37, 38, 148, 241–42
Nutrition, 30, 208–13, 217. *See also* Elimination; Intravenous (IV) hydration; Mouth care; Nausea; Swallowing difficulties.

O
Occupational therapists, 64
Odors, patient, 32. *See also* Bathing.
Oncology Nurses Association, 232, 238
Out-of-pocket costs, 50–51, 65
Ovarian cancer. *See* Alice Clark.
Oxygen, 230

P
Pain control. *See also* Ethical dilemmas, comfort vs. treatment; Medication; Pain medication; Palliative care.
and addiction, 232
and AIDS, 257–58
breakthrough, 230
by caregiver, 17, 86–87, 231–33, 238–40
for comatose, 233
environment and, 88, 235

Pain control *(cont.)*
  by hospice, 53, 54, 55
  hospitalization for, 5, 26, 37, 82
  by physician, 21, 60, 160, 231, 238
  resources, 238–39
  strategy for, 231–34
Pain medication. *See also*
  Medication; Pain control;
  Patient log.
  administration of, 21, 231–37
  alternatives to, 235–37
  overdose of, 86
  side effects, 232, 245–47
Palliative care, 4, 8, 25, 40, 48, 53.
  See also Ethical dilemmas,
  comfort or treatment; Pain
  control.
Patient log, 94–98
Perineal care, 11, 150, 203
Peripheral intravenous catheter
  (PIC line), 229
Personality changes, xix
Pharmacists, 64
Phased discharge, 26
Physical therapists, 64, 204, 220
Physicians
  and caregiver, 18, 21–22, 24, 60–62
  and death certificate, 248
  home care agency, 34, 58–60, 64, 68–69, 248–49
  home visits by, 54, 61–62
  hospice, 48, 53–54, 62, 248–49
  and pain control, 60, 69, 82, 86, 231, 238
  reimbursement for, 54, 58–59
  selection of, 61–62, 98n
  and terminal care, 21–22, 60–62
Physician-assisted suicide, 158
Pneumatic lifts, 31, 81, 220
Port, 229

Posey jacket, 219
Professionals, types of. *See also*
  Formal support.
  equipment technicians, 31
  lab technicians, 64
  occupational therapists, 64
  pharmacists, 64
  physical therapists, 64, 204, 220
  psychiatrists, 64, 92
  recreation therapists, 64
  respiratory therapists, 19
  social workers, 7, 47, 64, 123
Prospective payment system, 5
Protease inhibitors, 170, 251
Psychiatrists, 64, 92
"Pulling the plug," 4, 83. *See also*
  Ethical dilemmas.
PWA (People with AIDS). *See*
  AIDS.

Q
Quality of life, 29, 37, 47, 56, 98–100, 127
Quinn, Lawrence, xix, 16
Quinn, Martha (caregiver), 16, 114, 139–40

R
Recreational therapists, 64
Rectal tube, 217. *See also* Diarrhea.
Rehospitalization. *See also* Respite.
  and life support, 40–41
  process of, 39
  reasons for, 10, 36–39, 82–83, 152
Relaxation, 223, 235–37
Respiratory therapists, 19
Respite
  children as, 139
  hospitalization for, 5, 10, 42–43, 52, 55
  Medicare for, 36

reasons for, 10, 36–38
short breaks as, 33, 141–42
types of, 42, 46, 105, 106, 114–15
Restraints, 218–20
Roehm, Carl, xix, 16
Roehm, Mary (caregiver), 16, 108, 120, 185

S
Seizures, 24, 174, 231
Sexuality, 161, 207–8
Side effects. *See* Adverse drug reactions.
Skin care. *See* Decubitus ulcer.
Sleep
aids, 223–24
caregiver's, 10, 36, 52, 129–31, 223
disorders, 8, 10, 38, 52, 223–24
fear of, 10, 223–24
impending death and, 153
pills for, 223–24
Smith, Joyce, xix–xx, 15, 16, 76–77, 170–72. *See also* Klein, Lucinda (caregiver).
Social support. *See* Informal support.
Social workers, 7, 47, 64, 123
Spiritual support, 46–47, 104, 108–10, 148
Stead, Dorothy, xx, 16, 172–74
Stead, Joe (caregiver), 16, 63, 80, 129, 150, 172–74, 209, 211
Steiner, Bonnie (caregiver), 16, 43, 103, 112, 119–20, 122, 125, 149, 174–75, 186–87, 192–93
Steiner, David, xx, 16, 174–75
Suctioning, 19, 31, 56, 80, 149
Suicide, xx, 12, 157–58, 170–72, 192, 242
Supplies, 30
Support groups, 50–51, 143–44

Suppositories, 29, 165, 234
Swallowing difficulties. *See also* Mouth care; Nutrition.
causes of, 27, 29
with medication, 19, 27–29, 56, 165, 212, 226
near death, 84, 154, 162, 165
Sweet, Laura (caregiver), 16, 45, 72–73, 74, 81, 82, 92, 106, 107, 109, 115, 122, 129, 137, 141, 142, 143, 147, 148, 152–53, 190, 225. *See also* Lane, Anthony.

T
Testicular cancer. *See* John Wright.
Texas catheter, 216
THC (tetrahydrocannabinol), 211, 214
Transfers
from bed to chair, 220–22
from bed to tub, 236
from hospital to home, 34–35
Tremors. *See* Seizures.
Turning, in bed, 37, 202, 204–7. *See also* Decubitus ulcer.

U
Urinal, 216

V
Venous access device, 229
Visitation, 33, 89–92, 104–5, 164
Visualization, 236–37

W
Will, preparation of, 182, 194–95. *See also* Living will.
Withdrawal of life support. *See* Life support systems.
Wolf, Helena (caregiver), 12–13, 16, 34, 36, 52, 60–61, 72, 81–82, 88–89, 91, 104, 107, 117–18,

Wolf, Helena (caregiver) *(cont.)*
    121–22, 126, 127, 128, 129, 133,
    136, 140–41, 145–46, 175–77,
    190–92, 198, 225–26
Wolf, Herbert, xxi, 16, 175–77
Work, 51, 146–48
Wound dressing, 44, 82, 204

Wright, Helen (caregiver), 16, 55–
    56, 103, 107, 108, 128, 132, 148,
    150, 177–80, 188, 211, 219
Wright, John, xxi, 16, 177–80

Y
Yoga, 131, 241

ANDREA SANKAR is an associate professor in the Department of Anthropology at Wayne State University in Detroit, where she is director of the Medical Anthropology Program. She specializes in the areas of HIV, aging, death and dying, and home care, on which she is widely published. Her works include *The Home Care Experience* and *Qualitative Methods in Aging Research*, both with Jaber Gubrium.

Andrea Sankar has done extensive fieldwork in Hong Kong, where she lived in a Buddhist nunnery while studying aging. She has done research on caring for Alzheimer's disease patients at home, medical technology in the home, home visits by physicians, and the impact of the prospective payment system on home care. With Mark Luborsky, she is founder of the Critical Empiricism Group in Gerontology. Her current work is in community care for people with HIV/AIDS.

Dr. Sankar was a nominee for the 1991 Margaret Mead award for *Dying at Home* and was the 1994 recipient of the Wayne State University Mentor Award. In 1995 the *Detroit News* named her "Michiganian of the Year" for her work in HIV/AIDS. In 1997 she was appointed a permanent member of the study section at the National Institute of Mental Health. She lives in Ann Arbor, Michigan, with her daughter.

Library of Congress Cataloging-in-Publication Data

Sankar, Andrea.
    Dying at home : a family guide for caregiving / Andrea Sankar. — Rev. and
updated ed.
       p.   cm. — (A Johns Hopkins Press health book)
    Includes bibliographical references and index.
    ISBN 0-8018-6202-7 (alk. paper). — ISBN 0-8018-6203-5 (pbk. : alk. paper)
    1. Terminally ill—Home care. I. Title. II. Series
R726.8.S26   1999
362.1'75—dc21   99-14613
                                                             CIP